POLICING PAIN

Policing Pain

The Opioid Crisis, Abolition,
and a New Ethic of Care

Kevin Revier

NEW YORK UNIVERSITY PRESS
New York

NEW YORK UNIVERSITY PRESS
New York
www.nyupress.org

© 2025 by New York University
All rights reserved

Please contact the Library of Congress for Cataloging-in-Publication data.

ISBN: 9781479828937 (hardback)
ISBN: 9781479828951 (paperback)
ISBN: 9781479828982 (library ebook)
ISBN: 9781479828975 (consumer ebook)

New York University Press books are printed on acid-free paper, and their binding materials are chosen for strength and durability. We strive to use environmentally responsible suppliers and materials to the greatest extent possible in publishing our books.

The manufacturer's authorized representative in the EU for product safety is Mare Nostrum Group B.V., Mauritskade 21D, 1091 GC Amsterdam, The Netherlands. Email: gpsr@mare-nostrum.co.uk.

Manufactured in the United States of America

10 9 8 7 6 5 4 3 2 1

Also available as an ebook

This book is dedicated to those who have passed away as a result of incarceration, policing, or overdose: in their memory, we continue to fight.

CONTENTS

Introduction

A Shifting Drug War

A young white woman stepped to the podium of a community theater, located in a deindustrialized city in upstate New York. Laura (pseudonym), a recent drug court graduate, offered a pivotal moment in her recovery:

> I was caught and arrested. As I was handcuffed, the officer told me he felt bad when he put the handcuffs over my track marks [from intravenous heroin use]. He somehow knew I just had a baby. He said, "[Laura], this isn't the life for you, and you know it. This is your second chance, change or die. Come to the department and show your arms healed from the track marks."
>
> After five months, I regained custody. This is proof that God works in mysterious ways. The arrest saved my life. Angels come in black and blue clothes.[1]

Laura is one of the many people affected by opioids in the United States. In 2017, over seventy thousand individuals died from drug overdose, surpassing peak annual deaths from guns, vehicle accidents, and HIV/AIDS.[2] While the overdose rate dipped to sixty-seven thousand in 2018, it rose to seventy thousand in 2019 and to ninety-one thousand in 2020, in part due to the COVID-19 pandemic. Since 2021, it has remained over one hundred thousand each year.[3] Opioids have played a major role in the death toll, including OxyContin in 1999, heroin in 2010, and fentanyl in 2013.[4] Journalists have documented the impact of opioids in small towns and rural regions facing job loss, in suburbs populated by people who are white and middle class, and in urban centers where residents have been found overdosed "in public restrooms, in parks, and under bridges."[5] News outlets have reported on opioid-dependent newborns, drugged driving, and financial costs, with federal spending amounting to $2.5 trillion from 2015 to 2018.[6] The opioid overdose rate has been deemed a mass-casualty event, an epidemic, a *crisis*.

As evident in Laura's story, public officials have taken a different approach from the tough-on-crime drug war strategy of the past fifty years. When the Centers for Disease Control (CDC) declared opioid overdose an epidemic in 2011, Drug Czar Gil Kerlikowske proclaimed, "As someone who has spent their entire career in law enforcement, I know we cannot arrest our way out of the drug problem." In 2016, President Barack Obama signed the Comprehensive Addiction and Recovery Act (CARA), which added $1.1 billion for drug treatment and research as well as $500 million for overdose prevention, including for the distribution of the opioid-reversal drug Naloxone (brand name Narcan).[7] In 2017, President Donald Trump declared the opioid overdose rate a public health emergency, and the 2018 First Step Act expanded access to medication-assisted treatment (MAT) in federal prisons.[8] President Joseph Biden heralded a federal recovery agenda to provide treatment support for people with substance use disorder (SUD), increase economic opportunities for those in recovery, and improve access to prison-based MAT.[9] In New York, which has exceeded the national average in fatal overdoses, public officials have also promoted treatment and criminal justice alternatives, including police-, court-, and incarceration-based treatment services.[10]

While some has changed, much has remained the same. Laura was, after all, arrested, incarcerated, and processed in a *criminal* court, with the threat of future incarceration always present. Opioid possession remains a federal and statewide criminal offense. In New York, simple possession of heroin can lead to one year in jail and up to a $1,000 fine. Depending on the quantity of a controlled substance, one can receive an eight- to twenty-year prison sentence with up to a $100,000 fine.[11] Counties across New York State have also invested in jail construction and expansion, particularly in rural and low-income areas hit by staggering overdose rates.[12] Perhaps Laura's story represents not a rolling back of the drug war but a *shifting* drug war, based on a widespread mixture of medicalization and criminalization for criminal justice investment, particularly in response to an opioid crisis that continues to capture the nation's attention.

In what ways has the opioid crisis contributed to carceral investment, even as politicians have declared, "We can't arrest our way out of this"? How, in a time of opioid crisis, has the criminal legal system—which is primarily composed of police, courts, and incarceration facilities—expanded in rural and deindustrialized areas?[13] In what ways do stories of addiction, treatment, and recovery bolster mass incarceration, mass policing, and mass supervision? To explore these questions, I spent two and a half years conducting fieldwork, from December 2017 to May 2019, in the Southern Tier of New York, a region impacted by deindustrialization, mass incarceration, and overdose crisis.

From Shoes to Shackles

The seat of Broome County, Binghamton, is located at the confluence of the Chenango and Susquehanna Rivers in central New York State. In 1786, the wealthy Philadelphian William Bingham bought 32,620 acres of land from New York State, land occupied by the Onondaga Nation.[14] On July 4, 1800, Bingham offered the land speculator Joshua Whitney Jr. a grant "to plan a community in which trades, industries and arts would flourish."[15] On December 3, 1855, the New York State legislature divided the Town of Chenango, which created the Town of Binghamton.[16] The 1837 construction of the Chenango Canal was, while a financial bane for the state, instrumental for Binghamton's early development.[17] It was "an anchor for the city's commercial center," as it "drew industries, businesses, and people."[18] Binghamton subsequently developed as a shipping and processing center for extractive industries, such as lumbering.[19] In the mid-nineteenth century, the city turned to cigar manufacturing and became the second largest producer in the country by the 1870s and 1880s.[20] Economic growth in Binghamton did not reach its apex, however, until Henry B. Endicott and George F. Johnson's late nineteenth-century founding of the Endicott-Johnson Shoe Company, or "E-J" for short.[21]

"Which way E-J?" asked thousands of immigrants from southern and eastern Europe seeking work. By the late 1930s, the company ran twenty-nine factories in the "triple cities" of Binghamton, Johnson City, and Endicott. By 1920, E-J had employed over twenty thousand people and, by the mid-1940s, was selling fifty-two million pairs of footwear annually, including business, sporting, and outdoor shoes as well as combat boots during World War II.[22] Staunchly antiunionist, Johnson built what he deemed an industrial democracy, offering "cradle to grave" employment, housing, and health care. The company maintained a bowling alley, athletic team, hospital, theater, library, golf course, pool, farmers' market, and six carousels that remain free to ride today. Further bolstering economic growth, in 1911 the industrial giant International Business Machines Corporation, or IBM, was founded in Endicott.[23] By the 1960s, IBM "was producing 70 percent of the world's computers and 80 percent of those used in the United States."[24]

Like so many cities in the rust belt, growth would not last. E-J was unable to compete in the current global economy.[25] Employment and employee benefits declined in the 1960s and 1970s, and the company shuttered its doors in 1998. IBM outsourced and left in 2002. The defense industry maintained Broome County through the 1980s. Yet, with the federal implementation of NAFTA, the remaining industrial base was decimated.[26] The city initiated several revitalization projects, such as investing in Binghamton University and utilizing a state-sponsored grant, Restore NY, to create "shovel ready" lots for private development.[27] Such investment, however, would not bring desired prosperity.[28] Homelessness more than doubled between 2010 and 2020, and the poverty rate was 50 percent above the national average by 2023; it was twice the national average for Black and Hispanic residents.[29] Newspaper headlines bemoaned, "Memories of Busier Times in Binghamton," "Hometown Isn't What It Used to Be," and "Can't We Just Make Binghamton Greater?"[30]

Along with small-town, deindustrialized, and rural areas dotting the US, Broome County turned to the criminal legal system.[31] Jails offer a pathway for revenue generation by housing federal and state incarcerated people and immigrant detainees and by contracting with private providers for health care, food, and communications.[32] While certainly not an economic panacea, criminal justice jobs offer decent pay, health benefits, and a pension.[33] In 2014, the county passed a $6.8 million jail expansion that converted a gymnasium into housing for incarcerated women, added a "state-of-the-art medical unit," and allotted thirteen new correctional officer positions.[34] From 2012 to 2023, the

Broome County Sheriff's Office budget increased from $29.1 to $42.8 million, which was nearly 10 percent of the county's operating budget. Those same years, the District Attorney's Office budget increased from $2.5 million to $4.2 million, and the Probation Office budget grew from $2.6 million to $4 million. The Public Defender's Office budget increased from $2 million to $2.3 million, although this was less funding in proportion to the county budget.[35] On top of this, funding for the Binghamton Police Department rose from $10.1 million to approximately $13.7 million.[36]

Importantly, as with Laura's experience, officials did not advocate for criminal justice spending through strictly law-and-order rhetoric. Rather, they appealed to improved health care, particularly pertaining to the opioid crisis. Indeed, when I began early "development of this research in 2016, Broome County ranked third in the state for fatal overdoses.[37] In local news, the Republican sheriff, David Harder, claimed that the jail expansion would provide support for people with "heroin problems," stating, "with the type of people we're getting in the jail every day—suicidal, an awful lot coming in with heroin problems so they go through detox, and we're holding four or five at all times with hard mental problems—the additional space will give us more room."[38] In 2017, the Republican district attorney (DA), Steve Cornwell, initiated "Safer Streets. Brighter Future," which combined drug investigation with police diversion to place "addicts" into "long term treatment." The DA also promoted drug treatment court to "prevent future crimes by helping addicts address their addiction issues and avoid jail and a criminal record."[39] The Public Defender's Office maintained commitments to drug court programming and, in 2019 and 2020, recognized an "increased caseload due to [the] drug abuse/opioid epidemic and criminal activities associated with such." The Broome County Probation Department regularly pointed to "a more volatile probationer" with "serious substance abuse, mental illness, and general aggressive tendencies."[40]

Carceral investment did not mean an increase in county-based public health—but a centralizing of funds within the criminal legal system. From 2012 to 2023, Broome County's mental health budget dropped from $1 million to $742,605, from 0.28 percent to 0.17 percent of the total operating budget.[41] Public health funding decreased from roughly

$1.9 million to $1.8 million, from 0.51 percent to 0.41 percent of the budget.[42] The year that the jail expansion was passed, the county also closed its mental health clinic.[43] Such funding decisions made the criminal legal system the primary way to receive county-funded treatment and health care support.

In this regard, Laura's experience speaks to an amalgamation of carceral-treatment operations in the community: of a caring police officer, a disciplinarian drug court team, and a jail always present as a recovery-oriented punitive measure. To explore the impact of this carceral trend and how stories like Laura's bolster it, it is important to consider the role of policing, historically and today.

Policing Social Order

What comes to mind when thinking of police? Although answers may vary, police are dominantly viewed as crime fighters who ensure public safety. Yet, as critical scholars have shown, police do little to prevent crime or to address community harm.[44] Instead, as Mark Neocleous argues, police fundamentally fabricate capitalist social order.[45] Capitalism is a social form based on endless profit accumulation, grounded on labor exploitation.[46] Workers produce commodities for a wage, and commodities are sold by owners in a competitive marketplace.[47] Not just wage labor but capitalism has developed through unpaid women's household work, chattel slavery, and colonial conquest to accumulate land and raw material. Given its rampant exploitation, alienation, and endless drive for profits, capitalism is met with constant crises and resistance. Police subsequently, as Alex Vitale puts it, "suppress[] social movements and tightly manag[e] the behaviors of poor and nonwhite people: those on the losing end of economic and political arrangements."[48] As I review here, policing fabricates capitalist order not just through the work of uniformed officers but through soldiers, settlers, and slave owners, all of whom perpetuate state-sanctioned violence— which haunts the opioid crisis today.[49]

Police were essential in creating a class of European wage workers in the sixteenth century. Prior to capitalism's global dominance, peasants lived on monarchic lands under the king's authority and were made to pay money or a portion of their harvest to lords who monitored them.[50] While this was an exploitative relationship, peasants had access to land, tools, and collective space, called the "commons." The Enclosure Movement privatized this land, turning small plots into large estates. Peasants were left, as the English farmer, journalist, and pamphleteer William Cobbett observed, "ragged as colts and pale as ashes."[51] Peasants moved to cities to work in factories, lest they starved to death. Yet, starvation was not always enough, so criminal laws prodded their movement from the field to the factory. A 1530 English law imposed whipping and imprisonment for "sturdy vagabonds," and a 1547 statute condemned idlers to "become enslaved, whipped, chained, and branded with the letter V on their breast."[52] English convicts, vagrants, and beggars were also sent to colonial America and were exploited through debt bondage; many were worked to death.[53] Simultaneously, women, who previously served as healers, midwives, and herbalists, were disciplined into unpaid household labor through campaigns of terror, such as the witch hunts.[54] In short, the peasant was policed out of the laborer.[55]

The development of capitalism relied on chattel slavery, tying together police, planters, and white settlers who transported, sold, and surveilled enslaved Africans made to work on plantations.[56] Slave codes, which had their blueprint in the Caribbean, maintained control of the enslaved.[57] New York slave laws restricted enslaved people from gathering in groups larger than three, banned the owning of land by free Black people, mandated that enslaved people fourteen years or older were required to carry a lantern if they went out after dark, and permitted the torturing and killing of "any slave who murders" or "plots with others to murder" their master.[58] Police acted as armed slave patrols. They surveilled rural roads to prevent escape and monitored enslaved people working off plantations, who could commingle with free Black people.[59] Slave laws also made it compulsory for whites to guard escape routes and to return escapees.[60] The Fugitive Slave Acts of 1793 and 1850 mandated Northern free states return escapees and fined those who assisted in their escape. Slave laws, thus, ensured that white settlers *acted as police* through the delegation of state violence.[61] Slave catchers, as Deirdre Cooper Owens writes, not only were motivated by money but "also performed a civic duty to a slaveholding nation that protected slavery at any cost."[62] The wage laborer was, thus, policed out of the enslaved African.

After the abolition of slavery in 1865, Black people continued to be policed as labor. The Thirteenth Amendment banned "slavery" and "involuntary servitude" yet permitted forced labor "as a punishment for crime whereof the party shall have been duly convicted." Slave codes turned to Black codes, which mandated that newly freed African Americans worked contracts and kept curfews. Punishments were also increased for crimes that African Americans were "likely" to commit, such as stealing pigs, and they "were more likely to be charged for minor offenses against 'good morals,'" such as "loud talking and being out at night."[63] As South Carolina Governor James Lawrence Orr proclaimed, Black people must be "restrained from theft, idleness, vagrancy and crime, and taught the *absolute necessity* of strictly complying with their contracts for labor."[64] Black codes filled jails, prisons, and convict camps, with the Black prison population outpacing the white prisoner rate.[65] Many were leased to planters who exploited them, with no financial incentive to keep them alive.[66] The newly freed were also met with violence by white vigilantes, such as the Ku Klux Klan (KKK), whose members monitored, killed, assaulted, and robbed Black families. Police at times joined the largely state-sanctioned violence.[67] KKK night rides turned into terror lynchings, lynchings into Jim Crow racial segregation (in which police enforced segregation laws and beat civil rights activists), and segregation into "colorblind" policies that have upheld concentrated poverty, organized abandonment, mass incarceration, mass policing, and mass supervision.[68]

Colonial conquest was essential for the exploitation of wage and nonwage labor. In the US, white settlers violently took over land they considered as previously unproductive. They regulated and killed Indigenous peoples through plagues and starvation, forced relocation, detainment, and "assimilation" in boarding schools, meant to "kill the Indian to save the man."[69] Indigenous peoples were raped, killed, and pillaged by state-controlled bodies and voluntary militias composed of individuals and families. The Virginia militia, as Roxanne Dunbar-Ortiz describes it, "was founded for one purpose: to kill Indians, take their land, drive them out, wipe them out."[70] Colonial governments even paid white settlers to retrieve the scalps of murdered

Indigenous peoples.[71] European artists and writers symbolized such conquest as a sexual encounter, depicting Indigenous women lying in wait for the "explorer standing erect, surrounded by ships and tools of navigation."[72] Policing has therefore been, as Sherene Razack puts it, "one site where white men and women (as well as those aspiring to whiteness), can enact racial hierarchy on behalf of the colonial state with impunity."[73]

Colonial settler violence became embedded in the National Guard, US Marines, and the Special Forces of the Army and Navy, which linked the state's war power abroad and police power domestically.[74] The Texas Rangers guided US Army forces into Mexico, "leaving a path of corpses and destruction to occupy Mexico City, where the citizens called them Texas Devils."[75] They also hunted Indigenous peoples accused of attacking white settlers.[76] When the US conquered the Philippines in the 1898 Spanish-American War (as well as Puerto Rico, Guam, and Cuba), the Philippine Constabulary acted as "a testing ground for new police techniques and technologies." The national police force developed close ties to monitor communities, erected telephone and telegraph wires to communicate intelligence, and utilized spies and agent provocateurs "to sow dissent and allow leaders and other agitators to be quickly arrested and neutralized."[77] The Pennsylvania State Police, which was created in 1905, adopted this model to counteract militant unionism by "putting down strikes, though often with less violence and greater political authority."[78] Indeed, domestic policing was meant to appear more legitimate than a standing army.[79] Nevertheless, as evident here, police and war power blur between settlers, police officers, and soldiers.[80]

Given this history, police largely protect *white capitalist order*.[81] Whiteness has been a key marker of citizenship in the US, with the 1790 Naturalization Act even limiting citizenship to white immigrants.[82] Race scientists attempted to naturalize white supremacy by equating whiteness, and thus Europeanness, with "freedom, civilization, rationality, and beauty."[83] Depictions of white freedom and civil order necessitated its counterpart: the racialized Other and, in particular, the African slave.[84] To make the enslavement of Africans appear natural, race scientists described them as animalistic, beastly, hypersexual, violent, savage, demonic, sluggish, thieving, and overindulgent.[85] Blackness would, in turn, become the "primary badge of slavery," as Saidiya Hartman puts it.[86] Hartman continues of the symbiotic relationship between the slave and the liberal bourgeois subject, "The slave is the object or the ground that makes possible the existence of the bourgeois subject and, by negation or contradistinction, defines liberty, citizenship, and the enclosures of the social body."[87] In this regard, racial capitalism requires racial policing, as police maintain capitalist order by appearing to be the "thin blue line" between white order and racialized disorder.[88]

Ultimately, as a manifestation of state power, policing—and its entailing violence—is employed not just by officers but by white settlers, enslavers, and militias to fabricate *white* capitalist order.[89] Policing, as Derecka Purnell reminds us, "is among the vestiges of slavery, colonialism, and genocide, tailored in America to suppress slave revolts, catch runaways, and repress labor organizing."[90] Policing relies on the politics of racial representation—particularly of white security to be protected from racialized insecurity. And, as security is never fully achieved, a permanent state of insecurity, or "ordinary emergency," is required to maintain capitalist racial order.[91] How has racial policing operated in the drug war historically, and how does it connect to drug war policing today?

Drug Policing and the Racialized Other

For a drug to be formally policed, it must be designated with a legal status. In the US, criminalized drugs include heroin, cocaine, and methamphetamine; medicalized drugs include Adderall and OxyContin; and legalized drugs include tobacco, alcohol, and caffeine. To be sure, the legal status of a drug does not mirror its chemical properties. After all, medically prescribed Adderall has much the same composition as more stigmatized and criminalized methamphetamine, and OxyContin is similar to heroin.[92] Drugs such as tobacco and alcohol, too, have proven quite deadly yet remain legal and widely consumed in the US.[93] For a drug to be criminalized, it must therefore be *labeled* as harmful and a threat to public order.[94] This labeling process has historically been through the connection of certain drugs with racialized outsiders—and, thus, is key for racial policing.[95]

The first federal prohibition policy was the 1914 Harrison Act, which regulated opium and cocaine.[96] Previously, both had been sold over the counter. Heroin was in cough syrups, and cocaine was advertised as a topical anesthetic and general cure-all.[97] With a rise of Chinese immigrant labor, reporters and lawmakers began to warn of Chinese opium smoking.[98] A *New York Times* article declared that Chinese immigrants were "addicted more or less to the habit of smoking opium."[99] The Chicago journalist William Rosser Cobbe wrote that Chinese opium smokers submitted to a "wantonness of desire." In contrast, he reasoned that Protestant white women who used morphine were "tied hand and foot by the physician," so they were "not morally responsible for their conduct."[100] The *Medical and Surgical Reporter* further cited racial mixing in opium dens, noting one physician who "witnessed the sickening sight of young white girls from sixteen to twenty years of age lying half-undressed on the floor or couches, smoking with their 'lovers.'"[101] The physician Samuel Collins reported the racial transformation of a Ms. Jones, who could be "anyone's next-door neighbor," but "she took crude opium and everybody knew it." This would make her appear stereotypically Chinese; as he wrote, "The opium was yellow, she lived in a yellow house, and she had a yellow skin."[102]

For cocaine, lawmakers, researchers, and reporters looked to another figure: the "negro cocaine fiend."[103] The doctor Edward Huntington Williams wrote in *The New York Times*, "The drug produces several other conditions which make the 'fiend' a peculiarly dangerous criminal. One of these conditions is a temporary immunity to shock—a resistance to the knockdown effects of fatal wounds. Bullets fired into vital parts, that would drop a sane man in his tracks, fail to check the fiend—fail to stop his rush or weaken his attack."[104] When speaking to Congress in 1910, Dr. Christopher Koch, the president of the Philadelphia Association of Retail Druggists, combined the cocaine fiend and the Black rapist myth: "The colored race in the South is very much perverted by cocaine and colored people seem to have a weakness for it and a great many of the southern rape cases have been traced to cocaine."[105] Based on the image of the cocaine fiend, police departments upgraded weaponry, and the Black rapist myth fueled vigilante terror lynchings.[106]

Six years after the Harrison Act, the federal government passed the Eighteenth Amendment, which banned "the manufacture, sale, or transportation of intoxicating liquors." Indeed, the roots of prohibition, and the disease concept of addiction more generally, began with Benjamin Rush's late eighteenth-century description of alcoholism as a disease of the will.[107] The entailing white-Protestant-led temperance movement adopted terms like "overwhelming," "overpowering," and "irresistible" to describe "the drunkard's desire for liquor."[108] With the twentieth-century rise of urbanization and immigration, the temperance movement began to support alcohol prohibition by pointing to consumption by Catholic immigrants.[109] Binghamton hosted a number of Women's Christian Temperance Unit (WCTU) chapters. The leader of the Broome County WCTU chapter, George W. Deland, complained of foreign invasion: "The foreigner who knocks and bewails at our doors to be admitted and then at his first opportunities violates the laws of this wonderful government ought to be obliged to pack his grip and return to the land from whence he came."[110] To this end, police and KKK vigilantes targeted bootleggers with "foreign sounding names."[111]

With the end of alcohol prohibition in 1933, another drug captured the nation's attention: cannabis.[112] During congressional hearings, Commissioner of the Federal Bureau of Narcotics (FBN) Harry J. Anslinger proclaimed, "Marijuana is the most violence-causing drug in the history of mankind."[113] He linked the drug to "Negroes, Hispanics, Filipinos, and entertainers" and noted that "marijuana causes white women to seek sexual relations with Negroes, entertainers, and others." Anslinger added for good measure, "Reefer makes darkies think they're as good as white men."[114] Connecting cannabis-induced violence to Mexicans, a Texas police captain asserted that the drug produces in them "a lust for blood" and "superhuman strength." He continued, "When they are addicted to the use they become very violent, especially when they become angry and will attack an officer even if a gun is drawn, they seem to have no fear."[115] A *New York Times* article, "Mexican Family Go Insane," featured a widow and her four children being "driven insane by eating the Marihuana plant."[116] The subsequent 1937 Marihuana Tax Act placed a federal tax on the drug and imposed prison sentences or fines for those who did not register.[117] Cannabis and heroin were further penalized with the 1951 Boggs Act, which established the nation's first mandatory-minimum sentencing for possession, and the Narcotic Control Act (1956) doubled mandatory-minimum sentences for sales of heroin and marijuana.[118]

The contemporary drug war has carried these racialized divisions—between white order and drug-induced, racialized disorder. When Richard Nixon was championing his law-and-order campaign, he referred to drugs as "public enemy number one." He spoke of violent protestors and criminals and of drug use spreading to the white suburbs, exemplified by the narrative of "the white girl from a 'good family' who experimented with marijuana and LSD and then became 'hooked on heroin.'"[119] The racial dynamics of his approach were evident in a now oft-quoted statement by his adviser John Ehrlichman, who admitted that the administration's goal was to get "the public to associate the hippies with marijuana and blacks with heroin."[120] In 1970, Nixon signed the Comprehensive Drug Abuse Prevention and Control Act, which created five drug classifications, including Schedule I drugs, deemed to have no medical value (e.g., heroin), and Schedule II drugs, deemed to have medical value (e.g., oxycodone and fentanyl). During his tenure, Nixon created the drug czar position to oversee drug policy as well as the Drug Enforcement Agency (DEA) to manage the drug classification system, and he led international drug war interdiction.[121] Indeed, Nixon's punitive approach was inspired by New York's 1973 Rockefeller drug laws, which included mandatory life sentences for selling drugs.[122]

If Nixon initiated the current iteration of the drug war, Ronald Reagan accelerated it in the 1980s. He stoked fears of Black drug use, while banking off a media frenzy over crack-cocaine consumption in urban areas. Journalists warned of crack babies, welfare queens, gang violence, and the drug spreading to the suburbs. *Newsweek* described crack as "the most addictive drug known to man," while claiming it causes "almost instantaneous addiction." It has "transformed the ghetto" and "is rapidly spreading into the suburbs."[123] Reagan, in declaring his tough-on-drugs ethos, claimed in his 1982 radio address to the nation, "We're making no excuses for drugs—hard, soft, or otherwise. Drugs are bad, and we're going after them."[124] And he did go after them. In 1986, Reagan passed the Anti-Drug Abuse Act, which determined a one-hundred-to-one sentencing ratio between crack and powdered cocaine and allocated $2 billion to antidrug enforcement. Subsequent federal laws drove this punitive approach, such as the Anti-Drug Abuse Act of 1988, the Violent Crime Control and Law Enforcement Act of 1994, and the Combat Methamphetamine Epidemic Act of 2005. Between 1980 and 1996, there was a tenfold increase in drug convictions, and by 2023, one in five people were incarcerated for a drug offense.[125] With the passing of the Rockefeller drug laws, New York's incarceration rate increased from ten thousand to seventy thousand over three decades, with roughly a third for a drug offense.[126]

To be sure, not just criminalization but policing has operated through the medicalization of addiction and treatment responses thereof. Indeed, the idea of confining those who are addicted to intoxicants dates back to the idea of addiction being a disease.[127] Rush recommended a "sober house" where drunkards could be granted "moral treatment."[128] The first institution designed to treat alcoholism as a disease, the New York State Inebriate Asylum, opened in Binghamton in 1867.[129] By 1900, there were over fifty such institutions operating in the US.[130] With the 1929 Narcotic Farms Act, the US Public Health Service opened narcotic farms in Lexington, Kentucky, and Fort Worth, Texas. Kentucky's "Narco" held patients seeking a "cure" as well as "inmates" convicted of federal drug crimes.[131] Nixon implemented a national system of methadone clinics, with the psychiatrist Jerome Jaffe leading the charge.[132] The 1986 Anti-Drug Abuse Act provided federal funds for drug treatment programs, and the 1994 Violent Crime Control and Law Enforcement Act allocated drug treatment funding in prisons.[133] When speaking to Congress in support of the 1994 crime bill, Senator Joseph Biden contended that prison treatment would "try to help [incarcerated people], try to change their behaviors," while ensuring that they are "away from my mother, your husband, our families."[134]

In this regard, policing is more than mere criminal, law-and-order suppression, but it operates through public health.[135] Indeed, the term "police" derives from the Greek word *polis*, which "was used to describe the group responsible for maintaining *health*, safety, and order in the community."[136] Like freedom, health is associated with white civil order.[137] After the abolition of slavery, for instance, African Americans were viewed as threatening the social body with "the vice and depravity presumed to reside in each and every drop of black blood."[138] Racial segregation was therefore meant to maintain the *health and security* of the nation.[139] Through the metaphor of the body politic, as Lambros Fatsis and Melayna Lamb remind us, the protection of the people therefore "consists of protection against threats to the state, which may be biological or viral but can be equally political, violent, or seditious."[140] Drug prohibition has been, in this regard, key for policing white national health from racialized disease and disorder.[141]

How has the framing of the opioid crisis as a public health problem—or what we may consider an *ordinary public health emergency*—contributed to racial policing? How do criminal and medical framings of addiction drive mass incarceration, mass policing, and mass supervision? In what ways do the intertwining legacies of settler colonialism and chattel slavery haunt drug policing today? It is such questions that I explore in this book.

Summary and Organization

What makes something a social problem? Social problems are not simply "out there." Rather, a certain condition, like the fatal overdose rate, must be *labeled* as such by claims-makers. Claims-makers are "the people who say and do things to persuade audiences that a social problem is at hand."[142] They include, but are not limited to, police, lawmakers, scientists, reporters, advocates, and community members, all of whom vie for public support on a hierarchy of credibility.[143] Claims-makers tell formulaic stories about the social problem that often involve stereotypical representations, such as of the "Chinese opium fiend" or "Negro cocaine fiend."[144] In chapters 1 and 2, I explore the social problem categories of the "opioid user" and the "opioid dealer," as offered in local and national contexts. Importantly, these categories do not represent individual people but are stereotypical representations that inform drug policy and are infused with historical representations of addiction and drug use, as I have outlined in this introduction.

In chapter 1, I recognize that the social problem group of the typical "opioid user" is of a medicalized white, middle- and lower-class person. While potentially humanizing, I argue that the medical framing of addiction as a disease tells of white racial degradation and, thus, is conducive for policing white racial order. Brain imagery technology and diagnostic criteria for substance use disorder portray white users as losing self-control, associated with white citizenship. Subsequent reporting documents whites as transforming into criminals and metaphorical beasts, zombies, and slaves, all associated with racialized Otherness.[145] For low-income whites, medicalized despair discourse incorporates images of poor and working-class white degradation, disease, and disorder.[146] Thus, medicalized addiction discourse presents a symbolic contrast between white order and racialized disorder at the site of the "white addict," in turn legitimizing police intervention through drug suppression *and* treatment.[147]

In contrast to the "opioid user," the social problem category of the "opioid dealer," as I offer in chapter 2, is of a racialized outsider and, within the New York context, a Black urban outsider in particular, who is deemed to threaten the white upstate community; this is despite that drug dealing generally occurs across racial lines.[148] I identify three dealer tropes: the dealer-as-outsider, who invades white space; the dealer-as-greedy-profiteer, who preys on white addiction; and the dealer-as-violent, who maliciously cuts drugs with fentanyl and engages in gang-related conflict. These tropes reinforce what Katherine Beckett refers to as the "myth of monstrosity," as they envision people who deal drugs not as responding to socioeconomic circumstances but as inherently violent, malicious, and evil.[149] The social problem category of the "opioid dealer" subsequently animates police suppression through drug raids, arrests, and expulsion.

In chapters 1 and 2, I recognize a racialized user/dealer divide. The "opioid dealer" is an outsider who is "*in* society but not *of* it" and is met with calls for exclusion. On the other hand, the "opioid user" is an insider who is "*of* society but not *in* it" and is met with calls for inclusion, albeit through criminal justice intervention.[150] Both types of social problem groups bolster the criminal legal system in a time of opioid crisis, even as politicians have declared, "We can't arrest our way out of this." What do such criminal-justice-based treatment initiatives look like?

In chapter 3, I consider the implementation of two police diversion programs, Police Assisted Addiction Recovery Initiative (PAARI) and Law Enforcement Assisted Diversion (LEAD) in New York State's Broome and Tompkins Counties, respectively. I detect elements of what I refer to as policing treatment, in which police employ medicalized addiction rhetoric to act as treatment gatekeepers. In chapter 4, I observe the local drug treatment court. I examine how therapeutic surveillance, which blends care and control, is rationalized through the courtroom construction of a drug court narrative identity. Drug court participants are made to identify as either a "recovering addict," associated with white civil order, or a "criminal addict," associated with racialized disorder. Such surveillance and subject making further entrench treatment within criminal courts. In chapter 5, I analyze popular narratives that frame jails as caring treatment providers. Contra these stories, I document carceral harms experienced by formerly incarcerated interviewees to argue that, despite some treatment support, jails are fundamentally places of degradation and dehumanization.[151] Taken together, carceral treatment programs produce the *treatable carceral subject* as someone who is subjected to the *care* and *control* of the carceral state, with the state appearing as "treatable" from the ills of the drug war past; it is a *treatable carceral state* filled with caring cops, courts, and cages.[152]

In observing the social problem construction of the opioid crisis, I utilize what I refer to as addiction politics. While "narcopolitics" refers to governance through drug possession, with the idea that those who possess and use drugs are doing so by exercising free will, much drug policy is based on the concept of addiction, a concept that is only made sensible within a social context.[153] Within racial capitalism, addiction is a proxy for threatened white racial order, which is characterized by freedom, health, rationality, and security.[154] White addiction narratives, which tell of whites metaphorically transforming into zombies, beasts, and slaves, therefore imagine the racialized insecurity to which whiteness is violently secured. Policing possession thus operates to restore white order by policing the racially *possessed*—marked by drug-induced enslavement and monstrosity.[155] With addiction politics, narcopolitics is necropolitics, as the condition of addiction is represented through the life-and-death-generating power of the caring and controlling state on the presumed life-and-death circumstances of the "addict" and, by proxy, the nation-state. Addiction discourse, to borrow from Sabrina Strings, is not about health but *hierarchy*, with addiction politics fought on what W. E. B. Du Bois referred to as the color line.[156]

The ongoing drug war, even with treatment investment, is *harm inducing*. Prohibition actively produces risks of overdose by shifting drug markets, by lowering tolerances for those who are incarcerated, and by moving funds from harm-reduction services to the criminal legal system.[157] Importantly, the politics of white racial resentment and racist fearmongering that drive the drug war kill whites, too.[158] If policing perpetuates overdose death, then we can say, rather grimly, that police power circulates through all the bodies—the veins, the lungs, and the nasal cavities—of those who overdose. Drug war is, ultimately, class war, and class war, as Ruth Wilson Gilmore reminds us, is "shaped by its modalities as race war, gender war, colonial war: the war of racial capitalism against all."[159]

Given the failure of carceral care to address the socioeconomic conditions that drive overdoses, I recommend in the conclusion a new ethic of care: abolitionist care. Abolitionists focus on tearing down systems of oppression and building up communities through mutual aid, healing justice, and liberatory harm reduction.[160] I look to aspects of abolitionist organizing across local groups that I worked with during my fieldwork, namely, Truth Pharm and Justice and Unity for the Southern Tier (JUST). Local organizers, to be sure, were not monolithic, nor did they necessarily identify as abolitionists. Indeed, I do not recall ever hearing the word "abolition" in the context of organizing at the time. Yet, I interpret local organizers as having practiced abolition by, for instance, developing mutual aid and demanding disinvestment in the criminal legal system. After all, abolitionist care means, as Alexia Arani defines it, "reimagining and enacting care beyond carceral logics of surveillance, punishment, and abandonment."[161] Indeed, by participating in these efforts, I aimed for a disruptive ethnography, in which the researcher enters into the politics of meaning in the field for theoretical engagement and empirical investigation, while advocating for and with those who are directly impacted.[162]

Ultimately, this book is about how medical discourse in a time of opioid crisis has justified the policing of people who use drugs, placing them within a punitive apparatus that binds treatment providers, medical professionals, police, courts, and jails. In this regard, the drug war operates not just through drugs per se but through the concept of addiction, as a way of imagining racialized (dis)order, which is key for capitalism's exploitation, marginalization, and policing. Subsequently, through the ongoing drug war, the capitalist conditions that drive opioid overdose deaths—as stemming from neoliberal policy making for the deregulation of the pharmaceutical industry, deindustrialization and job loss, and criminal justice investment—remain unaddressed through a politics of medicalized (in)security that warrants ever more policing.[163] And, through the continuing drug war, the carceral apparatus expands, ensuring that fatal overdoses continue.

Beyond the Opioid Crisis

"Will Adderall Be the New Opioid Crisis?," a writer asked in *Psychology Today*.[164] Or perhaps benzodiazepines will be "the next opioid crisis," a health-care provider pondered.[165] To be sure, meth, a reporter noted in *The Press & Sun-Bulletin* (Binghamton, NY), was a growing scourge, writing, "With the national focus on the tragedy of opioid addiction and overdose deaths, another illegal drug hasn't received the attention. But the use of meth still is a scourge—and a growing one."[166] Even Ozempic, the diabetes-turned-weight-loss drug, has been warned to be potentially "the next opioid crisis."[167] It is apparent that drug scares will continue to be, as Craig Reinarman points out, a "recurring feature of U.S. society," whether it be alcohol, cocaine, cannabis, heroin, meth, or opioids.[168] And, in each scare, the machinery of the carceral state grinds, whether through therapeutic or punitive regimes, with the term "crisis" even arousing a need for policing to restore social order.[169]

I use the title *Policing Pain* to indicate ongoing policing through the criminalization of what are dominantly referred to as painkillers. Pain has also been a central theme of the opioid crisis, as OxyContin's initial distribution was driven by a "right to pain management" movement.[170] The medical industry polices pain, too, particularly when marketing, prescribing, and monitoring painkillers.[171] Certainly, policing is painful for those who are arrested, with tight handcuffs and shaky transportation to courts and jails, where the incarcerated face the pains of imprisonment.[172] And prohibition, too, produces the pains of social disconnection and organized abandonment within racial capitalism.[173] Yet, I would like to take the meaning of policing pain further. With federal spending on the drug war amounting to approximately $44 billion in 2023, policing, in the colloquial sense, *is a pain*: a persistent effort to control, eradicate, and dominate, with no end in sight.[174]

In a time of opioid crisis, it is imperative to disrupt this cycle. It is critical to place the opioid crisis within a larger framework of racial capitalism, policing, and drug war, from which drug representations and policies derive. I hope that by doing so, and by promoting abolitionist care against carceral care, this book aids in such efforts.

1

Medicalizing Our Way Out of This

Local officials surround the conference table at the Public Health Department for the weekly meeting of the Broome County Opioid Awareness Council (BOAC). The County Supervising Public Health Educator stands in front of a projector to introduce an Rx CDC (Centers for Disease Control) media campaign. The initiative is part of a NYS Department of Health (DOH) program, with Broome County receiving a $50,000 grant. We watch the video, titled "Christopher's Story," to which the group reacts positively. The campaign is as follows,

"Ann Marie's son, Christopher, was a great student and a gifted baseball player, and he was very close to his mother and sister. When he was 20 years old, Christopher was in a minor car crash and was prescribed opioids for back pain following the crash. Christopher's tolerance grew quickly, and he sought out doctors who would prescribe him more opioids. . . . Within roughly two years of beginning to use prescription opioids, Christopher overdosed and died at just 22 years old."[1]

Christopher's experience dovetails with that of many who have been prescribed painkillers, became addicted, and overdosed.[2] Stories of opioid addiction and overdose have been told in news reporting, in obituaries, and by lawmakers, both locally and nationwide.[3] While not mentioning the origin of his drug use, the local *Press & Sun-Bulletin* reported on twenty-six-year-old C.J., who fatally overdosed on March 8, 2016. The coverage spoke of his culinary talents, musical abilities, and "gentle spirit." "He was just a really loving kid," his mother told the journalist.[4]

While such reporting has been key to bringing awareness to overdose deaths, those who have been featured often fit a common demographic: They are white. Reporting has abounded on a new white face of addiction. Consider ABC's "The New Face of Heroin Addiction," NBC's "Painkiller Use Breeds New Face of Heroin Addiction," Fox's "New Face of Drug Addiction," *Brava*'s "The Faces of Opioid Addiction," *Rolling*

Stone's "The New Face of Heroin," and *People*'s "Faces of an Epidemic," which listed "newlyweds, honor students, and executives."[5] Certainly, whites have been prescribed opioids at a rampant rate, and this has contributed to a spike in fatal overdoses.[6] Nevertheless, the popularized new face of addiction overlooks the overdose rate among Black, Latinx, and Indigenous groups, and it presumes that whites indeed do represent a *new* face of addiction, despite historically using drugs at a similar rate as people of color, if not at a higher rate.[7] Ultimately, the new white face of addiction *whitewashes* the opioid crisis.[8]

Scholars and reporters have argued, in turn, that the white medicalization of addiction as a disease has led to a gentler war on drugs.[9] This has historical precedent. As outlined in the introduction, in the early twentieth century Protestant women morphine users were considered by the Chicago journalist William Rosser Cobbe to be "tied hand and foot by the physician." Unlike Chinese opium smokers, they were considered as not "morally responsible for their conduct."[10] When white heroin use grew in the 1990s, President George H. W. Bush declared it the "decade of the brain" and cited the importance of neuroscience for "our war on drugs."[11] With the recent wave of white overdose deaths, Drug Czar Gil Kerlikowske stated in 2011, "Drug policy reform should be rooted in neuroscience, not political science."[12] Similarly, the National Institute of Drug Abuse (NIDA) Director Nora Volkow and National Institutes of Health (NIH) Director Francis Collins have highlighted "the role of science in addressing the opioid crisis."[13]

Yet, while the stereotypical image of the "opioid user" may be a medicalized white figure, and this has led to progressive policies related to treatment, government drug takebacks, and expanded naloxone access, I argue in this chapter that the social problem construction of medicalized white drug use, in reporting, research, and advocacy, evokes racialized disorder.[14] In particular, medical social problem stories tell of racial degradation from addiction, that of white opioid users transforming from law-abiding citizens into criminals and metaphorical beasts, zombies, and slaves.[15] These metaphors deem the "white addict" an object of insecurity, as they transgress categorical boundaries between white freedom and racialized enslavement and monstrosity.[16] For low-income whites, who are already symbolically associated with racialized Otherness, medicalized despair discourse further imagines collective drug-induced racial degradation—of a disordered class in disordered space. While helpful for some people to seek desired abstinence, treatment ultimately disciplines the racially disordered "addict" into proper white citizenship and, thus, white social order. To be sure, treatment is also ripe for criminal justice intervention, as seen in my interviews with local methadone and buprenorphine providers in the final part of this chapter. As such, police have arrested our way out of the opioid crisis by *medicalizing our way out of it.*

"A Scene from the Walking Dead": Medicalizing the *(Dis)*ordered Subject

The public event features a "Science of Addiction" presentation run by local advocates and prevention specialists. Tables are set up in front of a projector screen at the community prevention center. I am sitting next to a bookshelf with informational pamphlets and DVDs on "myths" and "facts" about drug use. An advocate speaks at the front of the room. She utilizes neuroscientific explanations to educate us on opioid overdose and addiction.

"Back when we were cavemen, we operated through primordial functions: food, sex, and water were wired into our pleasure center. Everything we did was based on pure function, pure drive. Heroin very quickly matches all other things necessary for survival. Suddenly food, water, procreation, nurturing, it'll take over the need for those. . . . Even caring for children is not as much of a priority anymore, as heroin serves that need. Heroin pretty much is the driving motivator to survive. The brain stops checking in with the judgment center, motivation center, and emotions. . . . It is totally in survival mode for the heroin. An overdose occurs when receptors become so full that the brain is unable to communicate to the body to breathe. This necessitates application of opioid-reversal Naloxone (brand name Narcan)."[17]

In this presentation, the advocate adopted a brain disease model by drawing on the brain's reward system regarding learning, tolerance, compulsion, cravings, withdrawal, and overdose. Indeed, local advocates, myself included, regularly employed medical explanations to offer drug-related awareness and reduce stigma; to support syringe-service programs, fentanyl testing strip distribution, safer consumption spaces, medication-assisted treatment (MAT), and naloxone access; and to discuss risks when mixing drugs, consuming alone, or using with a lowered tolerance.[18]

While medical explanations of addiction support lifesaving practices and can humanize people who use drugs, medicalization is also conducive to criminal justice intervention. The Prison Policy Initiative estimates that "more than 578,000 people (47%) in state and federal prisons in 2022 had a substance use disorder in the year prior to their admission."[19] On top of this, more than 44 percent of referrals to treatment are made through the criminal justice system.[20] As I review here, dominant medical framings of addiction, including NIDA citing addiction as a chronic, relapsing brain disease and the American Psychiatric Association's (APA's) diagnostic criteria for "substance use disorder," do not just report on addiction as a concept but convey a social problem formula story of white civil freedom and racialized enslavement and monstrosity.[21] Medical explanations in turn depict white racial degradation through the racialized *medically disordered subject*.

The brain disease model of addiction imagines the medically disordered subject in several ways. First, drug scientists focus on the negative aspects of drug use, even if they are, as the neuroscientist Carl Hart points out, "a minority of effects."[22] These effects are projected on brain scans, including with positron emission tomography (PET) and functional magnetic resonance imaging (fMRI). As such, they distinguish between the "normal" and the lit-up, drug-induced "abnormal" brain.[23] NIDA's "Drugs, Brains, and Behavior," for instance, shows an image of a "healthy brain" versus the "diseased brain" of a "cocaine abuser."[24] The "abnormal" brain is then described by neuroscientists as lacking willpower. Alan Leshner has explained that from prolonged drug use, "a switch is thrown," which makes use involuntary.[25] Similarly, Nora Volkow has argued that the "brain [of an addicted person] is no longer able to produce something needed for our functioning and that healthy people take for granted, *free will*."[26] Through the dominant neuroscientific perspective, drugs thus appear to turn the standardized (read: white) "normal brain," associated with liberal freedom, into the "abnormal brain," associated with racialized enslavement.[27] The diseased brain, in other words, represents a *diseased will*.[28]

Diagnostic criteria for SUD in the *Diagnostic and Statistical Manual of Mental Disorders*, 5th edition (*DSM-5*), also convey norms of white citizenship.[29] The first set of criteria includes "neglecting major roles to use," "social or interpersonal problems related to use," and "activities given up to use." While perhaps neutral at face value, within a capitalist system such criteria are bound up with notions of productive white citizenship that define the "rules," "activities," and "interpersonal relationships" that one must strive for. That is, such criteria are interpreted within "a culture attuned to the clock, a cultural frame in which time is viewed as a commodity that is used or spent rather than simply experienced."[30] The second set of criteria further focuses on a loss of self-control, citing "hazardous use," "using larger amounts/longer than anticipated," "repeating attempts to control use or quit," and "a lot of time spent using." The "addict" is therefore, as Helen Keane describes, "someone who has lost control over their desires and thereby over their life, as evidenced in their failure to meet work, family and social expectations."[31] The final set of criteria evokes physiological transformation related to "withdrawal," "tolerance," "craving," and "physical or psychological problems related to use." While ongoing drug consumption can produce physiological effects, such criteria imagine, as Suzanne Fraser and colleagues put it, "vivid signs of the physical otherness of the true addict."[32]

Metaphors expressed by reporters, such as describing those who are addicted as "beasts" and "zombies," further incorporate tropes of racialized Otherness. In *The Least of Us*, Sam Quinones employs neuroscientific explanations to describe drug addiction by focusing on dopamine release "in the brain's pleasure circuit known as the nucleus accumbens."[33] He simultaneously tells of drug-addicted whites, who he claims are affected "in the great majority," as transforming from law-abiding citizens into a state of criminality and beastliness: "Parents who'd imagined some glowing life script for their newborns were, as those kids reached young adulthood, confronted with lying, stealing, conniving children, their bodies occupied by some mutant beast. Then came a felony record. Suddenly parents were cosigning for apartments, driving their addicted beloveds, now thirty, to a GED class."[34] Through medical discourse, whites thus become "occupied by some mutant beast"; they are "lawless creatures" with whom, as John Locke put it in his 1689 *Second Treatise*, "men can have no society nor security."[35]

It is worth considering the anti-Black underpinning, not just of criminality, which has been so well documented, but of the "beast."[36] To justify the Portuguese slave trade in the fifteenth century, the chronicler Gomes Eanes de Zurara reported that Africans "lived like *beasts* without any custom of reasonable beings."[37] Dr. John Harvey Kellogg, of breakfast cereal fame, reasoned that alcohol intoxication turned its users into racialized beasts: "The South is for prohibition because it has been forced to recognize that given whiskey, the negro is made a *beast*. The white man intoxicated sinks low enough in the bestial scale, but not so low as the negro or the Indian."[38] The beastly nature of drugs thus threatens white health/security, with whites sinking on a "bestial scale" most associated with Black and Indigenous use.

The medically disordered brains and bodies of the "addict" are perhaps no more evident than with the drug-induced zombie.[39] In *Unstitched*, Brett Stanciu investigates the opioid crisis in Hardwick, Vermont. While highlighting the disease model of addiction in the text, Stanciu also quotes Vermont's Hardwick Police Chief Aaron Cochran describing the opioid crisis as a "zombie apocalypse": "I see the opioid crisis as a modern-day zombie apocalypse. Drugs turn addicts into people nobody knows. They don't even know who they are anymore themselves. They're willing to do almost anything to get that high, regardless of who they hurt. The consequences don't matter. Family members are not family members to them anymore."[40] Not just opioids, but Sam Quinones also cites P2P, "new meth," which he considers the "fourth wave" of the overdose crisis, as creating a drug-induced "caste of people" who appear zombie-like: "This new meth itself was quickly, intensely damaging people's brains. The symptoms were always the same—violent paranoia, hallucinations, figures always lurking in the shadows, isolation, rotted and abscessed dental work, uncontrollable limbs, massive memory loss, jumbled speech, and, almost always, homelessness."[41] A West Virginian storeowner described to Quinones that downtown Clarksburg looked like "a scene from *The Walking Dead*."[42]

Like the slave, criminal, and beast, the zombie is constitutive of anti-Black imagery. As Tiya Miles writes, "A zombie is a slavelike figure whose existence of void consciousness is one of walking death."[43] As Alfred Métraux put it furthermore, "The zombi's life is seen in terms which echo the harsh existence of the slave. . . . The *zombi* is a beast of burden which his master exploits without mercy, making him work in the fields, weighing him down with labour, whipping him freely and feeding him on mea- gre, tasteless food."[44] The zombie thus threatens white order through concerns of racial contagion. After all, "zombies can be anyone," even white people.[45] As such, claims by reporters, police, and writers that "every human brain has the capacity for addiction," "opioid addiction isn't, well, prejudiced, so to speak," and "addiction is an equal opportu- nity affliction" not only whitewash addiction, as they imply a deracial- ized white figure, but warn of a contagious outbreak.[46] As David Sheff cautions in *Clean*, "Your education, safe neighborhood, good income, strong family—whatever you think will protect you—guarantees noth- ing."[47] Such transformation reflects wasted whiteness, not merely in the sense of losing the benefits allocated from white skin but through a con- tagious physical *wasting away of white skin*.[48]

Overall, while the dominant medical framing of addiction may offer a somewhat humanizing representation of people who use drugs, such rhetoric bolsters policing's politics of (in)security by placing racial- ized order and disorder within the addicted white figure. While Robin Room acutely recognizes that the concept of addiction "allows the tell- ing of a gothic tale or horror story" without the need for "ghosts, devils, and zombies," addiction discourse certainly does rely on *metaphorical* ghosts, devils, and zombies.[49] Through addicted brains and bodies, the "human" is fabricated, as Tyler Wall puts it, "as a site of racialized in- security, always threatened by a regression to a violent, feral nature."[50] And, for the beast and zombie, all manner of police violence is deemed necessary, whether through coerced treatment or violent repression.[51] As brain science and diagnostic criteria largely focus on individual brains, bodies, and behaviors, what about medical explanations that incorporate social context?

"It's Our Culture Now, Taking Pills": Medicalizing (*Dis*)Ordered Space

The truth about these dysfunctional, downscale communities [white up- state New York, eastern Kentucky, or West Texas] is that they deserve to die. Economically, they are negative assets. Morally, they are indefen- sible. . . . The white American underclass is in thrall to a vicious, selfish culture whose main products are misery and used heroin needles. Donald Trump's speeches make them feel good. So does OxyContin. What they need isn't analgesics, literal or political. They need real opportunity, which means that they need real change, which means that they need U-Haul.[52]

So says the political commentator Kevin Williamson for the conservative magazine *National Review*. Here, Williamson taps into stereotypes of poor and working-class whites, as morally corrupt and prone to drug use. Charles Murray similarly employs the "culture of poverty" thesis, which was used by Daniel Patrick Moynihan to describe "Negro culture," when citing poor white values as an "alienation from the 'founding virtues' of civic life."[53] The "culture of poverty" thesis does much to represent poor and working-class whites as departing from the middle-class white citizen ideal. So too do widely mediated images of degraded poor white drug use, including reporters referring to OxyContin as "hillbilly heroin" or publicizing pictures of "meth mouth."[54] It is worth, too, considering how popularized despair discourse also represents white poor, rural, and working-class disorder.

In the best seller *Deaths of Despair and the Future of Capitalism*, the economists Anne Case and Angus Deaton account for an increased mortality rate from suicide, alcoholic liver disease, and overdose from 1999 to 2017 for whites who were between the ages of forty-five and fifty-four, did not have a four-year degree, and lived in rural and deindustrialized regions, with the largest increases in West Virginia, Kentucky, Arkansas, and Mississippi.[55] They argue that these "deaths of despair" among the white working class are a consequence of social disconnection from decades-long economic restructuring, which has resulted in stagnant wages, weakened unions, outsourcing, a precarious service sector, and an expensive and unresponsive health-care system.[56] This has been paired with widespread opioid distribution in these regions.[57] Economic loss has disrupted family, community, and religious cohesion, and despair has taken hold—and so has risky drug use and overdose.[58] The authors recommend health-care reform and economic transformation to "make sure that markets, trade, innovation and immigration work for people, not against them, or for some and against many."[59]

I do not take on Case and Deaton's empirical evidence, as has been done well by the economist Christopher Ruhm.[60] Rather, I consider why "deaths of despair"—as a "convenient label," as Case and Deaton put it—resonates publicly, as evident given that the book is a *New York Times* and *Wall Street Journal* best seller.[61] One reason is perhaps because the research highlights white death. Joseph Friedman and colleagues point out that a focus on white death in despair research reinforces a popular inattention to staggering Black and Indigenous premature death rates.[62] Despair research's focus on whites, as Helena Hansen adds, is furthermore "a racially coded way of humanizing addiction, of placing blame for addiction outside of the affected individual."[63] I complicate the latter point here by arguing that despair research resonates publicly, and particularly for a white and middle-class audience, because it suits mainstream representations of working-class white disorder—through imagery of spatial degradation, collective fatalism, crime waves, and a nostalgic rural gone by.[64] I thus consider what Michael Bell refers to as the *second* rural, composed of stories, ideas, and images.[65]

Despair discourse creates an image of white degradation by depicting the *transformation* of bucolic and prosperous white space into degraded, disordered space. As Case and Deaton describe, "Towns and cities in the heartland of America that used to produce steel, glass, furniture, or shoes, and that are fondly remembered by people in their seventies as having been great places to grow up, had been gutted, their factories closed and shops boarded up. In the wreckage, the temptations of alcohol and drugs lured many to their deaths."[66] Similarly, Sam Quinones reports on the 1993 closing of Dreamland, a swimming pool in "the blue-collar town" of Portsmouth, Ohio, that opened in 1929. Its closing was symbolic of the arrival of a new kind of Portsmouth devastated by opioids. He writes, "Two Portsmouths exist today. One is a town of abandoned buildings at the edge of the Ohio River. The other resides in the memories of thousands in the town's diaspora who grew up during its better years and return to the actual Portsmouth rarely, if at all."[67] While Case and Deaton speak of individuals acting within a geographical context, this context cannot be solely represented through numbers; despair must be *imagined* through *affective landscapes*, here in depictions of "abandoned buildings" and "gutted" factories "in the heartland of America."[68] Such imagery casts a larger framing of disordered social life so often depicted in representations of poor and working-class white space, from the coal mines of Kentucky to the rust belt of New York.[69]

The degraded rural is marked by a sense of collective fatalism. Fatalism is key in popular depictions of poor whiteness. Jack Weller's 1965 *Yesterday's People*, which portrays life in southern Appalachia, defines, as Edward Karshner observes, "Appalachians as a gloomy, fatalistic backward-looking people imprisoned by their own adherence to a life long gone."[70] In speaking to collective fatalism within the context of the opioid crisis, a West Virginian resident told the journalist Beth Macy for *Dopesick*, "It's our culture now, taking pills."[71] Indeed, Case and Deaton's underscoring of the *demand* side, versus the more plausible explanation of pharmaceutical *supply*-side availability for drug-related deaths, frames fatal overdoses as born out of self-destruction.[72] As Case and Deaton argue, "People who put themselves at risk of dying from the side effects of alcohol or drugs have already lost much of what makes life worth living, paralleling the loss experienced by many of those who decide to kill themselves."[73] It is, for the authors, "tempting to classify [all deaths of despair] as suicides."[74] In critiquing such representation, bell hooks has pointed out, "Rarely do intellectuals, journalists, or politicians . . . suggest by their rhetoric that one can lead a meaningful, contended, and fulfilled life if one *is* poor."[75]

The degraded rural is also imagined to be taken over by drug-induced crime. While Case and Deaton do not discuss crime trends, they apply a medicalized framework to explain that addiction makes people "lie or steal to protect and feed it."[76] With regard to property crimes, in the wake of OxyContin's release, police and journalists warned of a late-1990s crime wave in central Appalachia. A Virginia police chief, for instance, reported that "about 90% of all thefts, burglaries and shoplifting incidents in the area were linked to the OxyContin trade."[77] Similarly, a local police officer on a public education panel I spoke on stated that there had been an increase in drug-related burglaries in the area.[78] Certainly, some people who use drugs do commit crimes to obtain drug money. Yet, property crime rates have been largely overstated, as observed in Kenneth Tunnell's research and has been evident in Broome County.[79] Nevertheless, despair discourse suits an image of widespread crime through drug-induced disorder so often associated with the working class.[80]

Despair discourse imagines not only a degraded rural but also a bucolic and prosperous industrial past. While nostalgia can open critiques of present economic and social conditions, it also tends to create a distorted representation of history.[81] In Broome County, for instance, nostalgia largely bears on prosperity wrought by the Endicott-Johnson Shoe Company. It depicts an ostensibly secure, benevolent, white capitalist order, which, as Mary O'Donovan argues, "subsume[s] class conflict under community progress."[82] White nostalgia furthermore obscures histories of racial segregation and colonial settlement.[83] Nostalgia can also appeal to reactionary politics. In Donald Trump's 2017 presidential inauguration speech, he described "rusted-out factories scattered like tombstones across the landscape of America." This metaphoric construction implies, as Nancy Isenberg interprets, a call to "recover[] greatness" by "replenishing the strength of an all-American workforce, returning it to its accustomed (and deserved) position at the top of the food chain."[84] In turn, images of the bucolic rural and industrial past produce *nostalgia (in)security*, where the nostalgic past of *white order* is in a drug-induced—and thus racially degraded—decline.

To be sure, despair scholars like Case and Deaton do not explicitly espouse such imagery. In fact, they actively reject the idea of a dysfunctional white working-class culture and are critical of policies that cater to corporate profiteering.[85] Nevertheless, despair discourse resonates well with a middle-class white audience, because it suits the notion of poor, rural, and working-class whites as a *disordered class* in *disordered space*. And, to be sure, the insecure heartland/homeland must be protected.[86] Police then establish order, whether through drug suppression, arrests, or even public health. Indeed, while not discussed by Case and Deaton, there has been an expansion of prisons and jails in rural and deindustrialized areas marked by overdose deaths.[87] Treatment, as I explore in the next section, further operates to regulate medically racialized (dis)order—*it is policing*.

"The Law Was Still a Part of It": Treating the (*Dis*)Ordered Subject

"The West Virginia photographer Lori Swadley wanted to feature something other than overdoses," Margaret Talbot wrote for *The New Yorker*. "And in January 2016, she started on another quest to see and remember: she would photograph addicts in recovery." Swadley's project offers a hopeful image, not of drug overdose but of addiction recovery.[88] People in recovery have also taken to social media to share experiences and provide support. In the Facebook group of the nonprofit Faces of Opioids—Stories of Using, Death and Recovery, participants have uploaded recovery photos and supportive messages with hashtags such as #wedorecover.[89]

While recovery narratives are certainly empowering, recovery, like the concept of addiction, reinforces an image of white civil order and racialized disorder. The Betty Ford Institute defines recovery as "a voluntarily maintained lifestyle characterized by sobriety, personal health, *and citizenship*," and the Substance Abuse and Mental Health Services Administration (SAMHSA) lists four "major dimensions" of recovery: health, home, purpose, and community.[90] Akin to diagnostic criteria for SUD, these characteristics may appear neutral at face value, but they are within a capitalist system that values individual freedom associated with white citizenship, which is modeled after the "self-steering, autonomous and entrepreneurial" subject born out of the fifteenth- and sixteenth-century Protestant Reformation.[91] Addiction turns the free white citizen into a state of enslavement, associated with racialized disorder. As the temperance writer Nathan Beman declared in 1829, "Drunkenness is itself a disease. . . . When the taste is formed, and the habit established, *no man is his own master*."[92] Recovery and addiction are thus bound together, as depicted in before/after photos, the Dr. Jekyll/Mr. Hyde duality, and the master/slave relationship.[93] The ordered "recovered citizen" is, in short, the flip side of the racially disordered "addict."

Treatment subsequently acts to return the addicted racially degraded subject into healthy citizenship.[94] On July 25, 1933, President Franklin Delano Roosevelt wrote to the Lexington, Kentucky, Board of Commerce regarding the state's Narcotic Farm, "It is fitting the Federal government should dedicate this institution to the noble purpose of rescuing our fellow men from the *abject slavery* of the narcotic habit. In this institution the victims of the opium habit will be *restored to usefulness*."[95] Scott Vrecko furthermore deems medication-assisted treatments such as Naltrexone, which reduces cravings for compulsive behaviors, as civilizing technologies: They produce individuals who are "more responsible and more able to adhere to the duties, expectations and obligations of their families and societies. That is, a state in which individuals are better *citizens*."[96] Treatment thus operates through what Michel Foucault refers to as the "biopolitics" of health management, which includes disciplinary practices to manage the medically disordered subject.[97] In the following, I draw on interviewees' experiences to identify disciplinary aspects of outpatient treatment for methadone and buprenorphine.

Methadone treatment began in the US in 1947. Participation requires daily observation at designated facilities with observed dosing and drug testing.[98] Given these mandates, participants have described methadone clinics as "liquid handcuffs."[99] Patients, too, are viewed as "unruly" and "noncompliant."[100] Due to the drug's stigma, interviewee Hannah felt that her use affected her employment opportunities: "I applied for a job, and they asked me if I was on [methadone]. This is shortly after we [she and her boyfriend] got clean, and I wasn't on probation. I had no felonies or anything at this point. They needed to know what kind of medications I was on. I was on methadone at the time. They asked me, 'Well, what are you on that for?' And I said, 'Because I'm a recovering addict.' I got denied the job because of that." Interviewee Elizabeth was able to access methadone in jail, as she was pregnant. Yet, she was torn between the strict regimen and the whims of correctional officers:

Being on methadone every single Tuesday. I had to go to the clinic to get my stuff, and the jail would forget to put that in the computer. So, I would be sitting there waiting for them to call me down to leave, and one day they didn't call me down, and I go to the CO [correctional officer]. I was like, "Sir, I need you to go to the methadone clinic. I'm supposed to go at this time."

He was like, "I don't know what to tell you. They'll call you down if they—if you're going to go or not." And I'm like, "No, you don't understand." . . . I go every Tuesday, and he wouldn't listen to me, and I was like, "Okay, when is the sergeant coming in? I need to talk to him."

And he refused to call the guy. He was like, "He's busy right now. He's not coming." And I was starting to get really sick, because I didn't have this medication, and the sergeant came in like every hour, every two hours, I think, to do a check. So, finally, he came in, and then I went and talked to him, and I was like, "Can you please, like please"—I was starting to cry—"just go check? I'm not trying to waste your time." That's how you had to be if you wanted to get anything from these guys. You had to be extremely polite and try to appeal to their ego almost.

Unlike methadone, buprenorphine (brand name Suboxone) is provided by private physicians who have Drug Enforcement Agency (DEA) certification. Rather than going to a clinic daily, participants receive doses for at-home use. Access often requires cash payments or private insurance. Of note, buprenorphine patients are predominantly white, unlike methadone treatment, which skews toward people of color.[101] Paying cash to doctors made one participant feel as though he was still visiting "the drug dealer." Interviewee Nate stated, "You have to cash pay, these doctors. If you pay them a certain amount of money, they give you as much Suboxone as you want. It's crooked; it's a crooked business. It was like going to the drug dealer." While interviewee Sarah's provider did take Medicaid, she had to pay $300 for the first visit and $40 each week thereafter: "On the initial visit, you have to pay $300 cash. Then, every week after that, you have to pay $40. . . . Then insurance—my Medicaid covers my script. . . . Otherwise, I have to pay $11 per strip, and I have fourteen of them. So thank God that the Medicaid pays. That's the one thing. I know it sucks that I've got to pay for the doctor's visit, but it's the only way that I could get in because it's not readily available." Sarah also spoke of the long waiting list for her provider, adding, "I knew this girl a few years ago. She waited for a year. They literally told her, they're like, 'It's probably gonna be about a year before we can get you in.'"

Even with at-home prescriptions, many buprenorphine providers require on-site drug testing. This can have a chilling effect for clients. As interviewee Ron put it, "You gotta sneak in fake piss." While toxicology testing can be important for physicians to consider medication use, such testing can also be an adjunct to criminal-justice-based surveillance. Nate appreciated drug testing as a form of accountability, but he felt that being on probation hindered his recovery experience: "The doctor I went to, . . . he did it the right way. He drug tested me. He held me accountable, wanted me to work the program. That's what I would expect. And they would talk to me, but also they realized that probation was a part of it too. So it was like, the law was still a part of it. I feel like if the law wasn't a part of what I was doing at the time, I would've had a good basis for recovery with Suboxone."[102] Thus, in methadone and buprenorphine outpatient treatment, there remains stigma, discipline, and criminal justice intervention.

Indeed, when I asked interviewees who use or had used drugs about a "solution" to the opioid crisis, many brought up accessible treatment services with no mention of the criminal legal system.[103] They suggested "a medical detox facility in this area with beds for long-term [treatment]," "a place where everything is all-in-one and included, . . . [with] family participation," "a long-term residential inpatient with more sober living," and a rehab that connects parents with children. "There's nothing like that," interviewee Kay told me. "You can't bring your kid with you to rehab. So that whole time, you're without your child. Your child's hurting 'cause they don't have you."[104] Yet, given the scarcity of services, the criminal legal system has often been the only way to receive treatment, wrapping in already strict methadone and buprenorphine providers. How such treatment operates is a primary focus in subsequent chapters.

Conclusion: Medicalization and Memorialization

> I am visiting Stephanie, whose son passed away from an overdose. We enter his bedroom. A quilt covers his mattress; it is made of shirts featuring popular rock bands. On his nightstand sits an urn of his ashes. "I'm telling you, the kid is here," she confides. "You probably think I'm nuts, but . . . I don't know. It's—he just—I'm telling you." We walk to the family's rock garden, built in commemoration; an emblem on a post in the garden signifies his organ donation, that, in his death, he preserved life.[105]

These experiences of loss are deeply meaningful. And medical terminology is a way for family members and friends to understand addiction and overdose and to advocate for loved ones. For Stephanie, offering Narcan trainings made her, as she put it in our interview, "actually feel like I'm doing something." For many, a switch does appear to be thrown within their loved ones or within themselves. Interviewee Pam made sense of her son's violent outbursts by reassuring, "I know that's not him." Kay, who had been sober from opiates for six years, felt, "You initially make that choice, and then it's like something takes complete control, and you don't know how to do it without it."[106]

Medical explanations furthermore helped interviewees who use or had used drugs make sense of their experiences. Nate utilized a medical framing when explaining his addiction. At the age of fifteen, he was pre-scribed ninety ten-milligram Percocet pills after being hospitalized for a week for a ruptured appendix. As he reflected, "Just being medically pre-scribed something for an injury, it's something I never knew would hap-pen to me, and [it] destroyed me for almost six years." Elizabeth referred to her previous use of cocaine, heroin, and meth as "self-medicating" bipolar disorder and depression. Interviewee Paul also referenced his "addictive personality" to explain difficulty maintaining prescribed opi-oid use, a concept that, while scientifically specious, felt personally in-sightful for my own complicated relationship with drug use, as I discuss in the appendix.[107] To be sure, medical researchers have considered a variety of coexisting psychological, biological, and sociological dimen-sions to drug use and addiction.[108]

Nevertheless, the dominant medical disease framing of addiction maintains a binary between free white citizenship and racialized en-slavement/monstrosity.[109] As Kate Seear and Suzanne Fraser put it, "In-sofar as late modernity is marked by a cultural valorisation of agency, rationality, autonomy and choice, the *diseased* 'addict' evokes horror to the extent that s/he [/they] signifies disorder, chaos, lack of control, uncertainty and irrationality."[110] As such, the medical model of addic-tion is not necessarily destigmatizing. As Carl Fisher contends, "Biologi-cal explanations increase aversion and pessimism toward people with psychological problems."[111] Interviewee William, for instance, felt that even after seven years in recovery, he was not able to maintain a positive identity: "I want people to understand. I want people to know me. I want people to see who I am, and nobody did that, and still to this day, I have trouble convincing people that after seven-plus years of being into my recovery, I still have people thinking I'm on drugs right now."

Addiction stigma, then, is not the product of individual bias or abstract prejudice but is embedded within a cultural system predicated on notions of white order and racialized disorder.[112] Addiction, as a policing concept, relies on imagery of racialized enslavement and monstrosity configured on the white body. Blackness therefore acts, as Saidiya Hartman describes, as an "imaginative surface" that allows for "an exploration of terror, desire, fear, loathing, and longing" and here of addiction, recovery, drug use, and health.[113] To protect white order, racialized disease discourse justifies the exercise of state power, including "*violent practices* thought necessary to defend the body politic."[114] Anti-Black racist ideas thus *haunt* medical explanations of addiction and *animate* policing for all manner of coercion, including through public health and treatment.

To be sure, carceral treatment is one prong of the carceral state meant to reduce the demand side of drug use, as I will explore with police, court, and jail treatment. Before doing so, it is important to consider the social problem construction of the "opioid dealer" as a racialized outsider who threatens white community.

2

The Dealer Divide

After winning the 2015 race, newly elected District Attorney Steve Cornwell rented a billboard near Binghamton's baseball stadium. On it, he directs police who are poised to enter a residence. The text reads,

> WARNING: Drug Dealers don't get deals in Broome County. THEY GO TO PRISON!"
> "Get Out . . . Or We Will Take You Out!"[1]

As evident here, the imagined opioid dealer, like the opioid user, is a prominent fixture of the opioid crisis.

Unlike the opioid user, however, the dealer has been met with police repression. Police arrests of people who deal drugs have increased nationwide.[2] Lawmakers have enhanced penalties for drug dealing and have passed drug-induced-homicide laws that establish "criminal liability for individuals who furnish or deliver controlled substances to another individual who died as a result."[3] Moreover, prosecutors have utilized felony-murder, depraved-heart, and manslaughter laws to charge people who dealt a drug that resulted in a fatal overdose. At a news conference, Cornwell described overdose homicide investigation as a "common sense" approach, "We are going to go after (drug) dealers, and we might as well go after the dealers who are killing people."[4]

Animosity toward drug dealers is nothing new; they have long haunted the public's imagination.[5] The stereotypical drug dealer suits what Katherine Beckett refers to as the "myth of monstrosity," which is a culturally embedded and stereotypical way of viewing violence—and here of dealing—as the result of "fundamentally depraved and brutal people who cannot be redeemed."[6] After all, monsters are, as David Gilmore describes, uncontrollable and unruly. They "embody all that is dangerous and horrible in the human imagination."[7] To be sure, the designation of monstrosity, as with the image of the drug dealer, is racialized. The abolitionist physician James McCune Smith wrote in 1852 of the monstrous representation of Black people, "The Negro 'with us' is not an actual physical being of flesh and bones and blood, but a hideous monster of the mind, ugly beyond all physical portraying, so utterly and ineffably monstrous as to frighten reason from its throne, and justice from its balance, and mercy from its hallowed temple. . . . It is a constructive Negro, that haunts with grim presence the precincts of this republic, shaking his gory locks over legislative halls and family prayers."[8]

How has the racialized monstrous dealer been imagined during the opioid crisis? In this chapter, I identify three racially coded dealer tropes, as expressed by community members, public officials, and reporters.[9] The first is the dealer-as-outsider trope, which presents the dealer as invading white upstate New York communities. Second is the dealer-as-greedy-profiteer trope, which envisions the dealer as cashing in on white addiction. Third is the dealer-as-violent trope, in which the dealer is deemed to maliciously cut heroin with fentanyl and engage in gang violence—putting the police and public at risk. Unlike narratives of white addiction, which tell of monstrous transformation through drug-induced racial degradation, dealer tropes presume monstrosity as already inherent within the stereotypical Black and, at times Latinx, figure. The racialized user/dealer divide, in turn, calls for all manner of punitive responses, bolstering police power through treatment for users-turned-monstrous and suppression for inherently monstrous dealers. To this point, Black people are more likely to be arrested for drug sales, despite that whites deal drugs at similar rates.[10] Yet, it should be noted that, through the anti-Black construction of the dealer, whites are also caught in the carceral apparatus—making the drug war truly a war against all, built on the foundation of racial capitalism.[11]

Dealer-as-Outsider: "Peddling Poison in Our Community"

In a Town Hall, Maine Governor Paul Lepage informed of invading dealers, "These are guys with the name D-Money, Smoothie, Shifty, these types of guys. They come from Connecticut and New York, they come up here, they sell their heroin, they go back home. Incidentally, half the time they impregnate a young white girl before they leave."[12] Not so subtly, Lepage offered the dealer-as-outsider trope, of a stereotypical, racially coded, Black criminal who invades white communities and threatens white women, who are presented as an object of sexual voyeurism.[13] With this trope, drug use appears as exceptional in white spaces. The suburbs are where drug problems "couldn't happen" or are a "deadly secret," and rural drug use is set against the backdrop of an otherwise bucolic heartland.[14] Alternatively, drug problems appear the norm in urban areas, with the dealer violating racialized boundaries when traveling to rural and suburban spaces to sell to white consumers.[15]

In the Southern Tier, the dealer-as-outsider trope occurred in local reporting of dealers traveling from surrounding urban centers to the upstate community, with the words "upstate" and "community" coded as white space. For one case, a journalist reported of a Black woman from Queens and a white woman from Brooklyn transporting heroin and cocaine "into the community," and another article read, "Queens woman accused of supplying cocaine and heroin upstate."[16] A reporter also cited two Black men who "funneled thousands of dollars worth of heroin into the community."[17] Certainly, there are drug distribution lines that run from urban centers to various regions in New York State.[18] Nevertheless, such reporting suits a long-standing media trope of racial invasion. From an analysis of one hundred popular press articles between 2001 and 2011, Julie Netherland and Helena Hansen similarly identified fears of racial mixing. A journalist, for instance, cited the Queens district attorney renaming the Long Island Expressway "heroin highway," connecting "Queens, which has a majority people of color, to Long Island, which is predominantly white."[19] Coverage also documented whites traveling to urban areas, with the *Chicago Daily Herald* warning, "Suburban teens who fall into the trap of heroin use often drive to West Side . . . to buy the drug."[20]

Local officials also presented a community threatened by outside dealers. On July 28, 2016, District Attorney Steve Cornwell announced the county's first major drug kingpin case, Operation Get Money, which resulted in the arrests of seven people and seizure of twenty-seven hundred bags of heroin, with a monetary value estimated at $40,000, as well as an estimated $38,000 in drug proceeds.[21] He declared in local reporting that dealers "come and poison *our kids*": "This indictment right here should serve as a message for the people that want to come and poison our kids and ruin lives and destroy our future. We're done with you.

Broome County is done. We want them to get out, we want them to get the hell out of Broome County."[22] When supporting the drug-homicide statute Laree's Law, which was cosponsored by the local State Senator Fred Akshar, Senator George Amedore stated, "We need to take on the heroin epidemic from all sides and that includes properly punishing the big business dealers that are bringing this poison into our *communities*."[23] Although Laree's Law has not been signed into law, supporters have nevertheless played on the image of a victimized white insider, as the law was named after eighteen-year-old Laree Farell-Lincoln, who died from a heroin overdose. A reporter described Farell-Lincoln as "a golden girl, with wavy blond hair, wide green eyes, a dazzling smile and a carefree spirit that radiates confidence."[24]

Public officials also warned of international invasion in upstate New York. When referring to a rise in overdoses in 2019, Oneida County Executive Anthony Picente stated that "the continual flow of drugs into the country" is "happening here": "We cannot allow the continual flow of drugs into the country, especially fentanyl, which could be a reason for the spike that we're seeing. . . . This is one of those issues in which you look at it and you say, 'It can never happen here.' But it is happening here. As a national issue, sometimes we see things, certain things around the country, that raise concerns and it doesn't touch home. This one touches home very significantly." In the same coverage, Democratic US Representative Anthony Brindisi appealed to threatened upstate families. He stated in support of stronger border control, "Opioid addiction is tearing families apart in upstate New York and across the country, and we need to do more to stop the trafficking of these deadly drugs."[25] The national territory is, thus, deemed to be *terrorized* by foreign invaders, who are imputed here in a local context, as the international drug trade "touches home very significantly."[26]

The dealer-as-outsider trope produces (white) community ire toward those who are deemed to be racial outsiders. As George Lipsitz points out, "Shared cultural ideals and moral geographies based on a romance with pure spaces . . . fuel[] allegiances to defensive localism and hostile privatism."[27] Residents expressed dealer hostility in a variety of ways. A bumper sticker on the back of a truck read, "Shoot Your Local Heroin Dealer."[28] Mug-shot photos uploaded on the sheriff's Facebook page of two arrested Black men from Queens received "like," "laugh," and "angry" emoji responses. Commenters wrote, "GET RID OF THE SCUM," "Gotta love all the trash moving up from the city," and "Congratulations on the capture of these two, spreading that POISON in our towns."[29]

Hostility toward the imagined racialized outsider shaped everyday racism confronted by Black residents in the Southern Tier. Interviewee Niya shared her experience of being associated with what Elijah Anderson refers to as the "iconic ghetto": "I've been living in this area since 1997. I'm not from Brooklyn. I'm an army kid. I did not grow up poor, and I've heard, 'Go back to Brooklyn,' more times than I can actually count."[30] White college students' racist perceptions of dealers led interviewee Michael, a middle-aged Black man who grew up in New York City, to begin dealing drugs in the first place. As he recounted,

> I come up here back in the late '90s, and, believe it or not, I was invited . . . by people that lived up here. Somehow they had themselves a [drug] line from California. We met through [the university, which] used to hold concerts back then. They were actually students. They made a [drug] connection with one of the artists that was performing, and they called us [Michael and a friend], because they were under the assumption that being Black, that you automatically knew what to do with whatever, which I had no idea. You know, I'm thinking that I'm coming up just for another party, because this is what we did. We traveled, and we partied, and went out to campus, and it was fun to do that. We got up there, and they're like, "Hey, man, we got all this stuff. We figured you could help us do stuff with it."
>
> . . . They figured I'm from low-income housing—automatically that qualifies me to know exactly what to do with these types of things, which in reality I had no idea. The roughest thing I'd seen was marijuana, because my dad and my uncles, they were into it. But me, myself personally, I had no idea. . . . I'm thinking, "Okay, so now what do I do?" I either . . . look like a total moron and lose all type of credibility with these guys who think that I'm cool, or I just play into whatever it is. So I'm like, "Yeah, sure, no problem."
>
> And that's how I started. . . . They gave me a bunch of stuff, put me in my car, and sent me on my way back to New York City. I had literally no idea what I was doing or what I was going to do with all this stuff. So there, right then that shows you. No, it's not dealers from somewhere else . . . who come up here ruining this beautiful, pristine town. No, like,

these guys—I got my first [drugs] from a white kid up here, you know what I mean?

In our interview, Michael thus subverted the stereotype of the Black dealer by pointing to what A. Rafik Mohamed and Erik D. Fritsvold refer to as "dorm room dealers": common, underrecognized, and often white drug dealers.[31]

Dealer-as-Greedy-Profiteer: "You're Not Addicted, You're Just Selling to Make Money"

I was meeting with April at a coffee shop. She was a white mother of a child who struggled with opioid addiction. As I sipped on my regular caffeine-loaded coffee, she commented on dealers, "I think there are two types of dealers. I know that anybody who has an addiction will do anything they can to feed that addiction. It's like a compulsion. It's out of necessity. I think the vast majority of dealers are low-level dealers that are just dealing to support their habit, and I think that they should be dealt with completely differently than those who are intentionally bringing drugs into the community to profit off it and enslave our young people." April here adopted a popular distinction between two categories of dealers; there are those who sell from addiction and those who deal to make a profit.[32] The latter is a greedy profiteer who *enslaves* young people. The user-dealer, in contrast, is dominantly represented as white, medicalized, and an ultimately redeemable figure.

The redeemable qualities of the user-dealer are shown in mainstream journalism on white street dealers. In "King of Boise: The Life and Times of a Teenage Oxycodone Dealer," Joe Eaton reports on Austin Serb. After a lucrative period of dealing, Serb succumbed to OxyContin use. His use spiraled, which led to a stint in prison that was the catalyst for his recovery.[33] In *Dopesick*, Beth Macy reports on the West Virginian Spencer Mumpower, who, after escalating use, sold the drug that killed his classmate Scott Roth. He transformed from, as Macy puts it, a "private-school student to federal inmate."[34] The novelty of such drug dealing in the suburbs was evident in Macy's earlier reporting, when she wrote, "two suburban Roanoke families became enmeshed in a growing heroin scene that ended with one son dead and another bound for prison."[35]

The user-dealer contrasts with the for-profit dealer, who is coded as a racialized outsider. This was apparent in sentencing statements made by the Broome County judge Kevin Dooley for people arrested in Operation Get Money. Of the seven arrested, three were charged as directors or profiteers. Terrance "Money" Wise, a Black man, was considered the director of the operation.[36] When offering a ten-year prison sentence as per a plea agreement, the judge combined the dealer-as-outsider and dealer-as-profiteer tropes: "Heroin is a problem in this community and in other communities . . . and your involvement in this went well-beyond just to support your own (drug) habit. . . . Next time, if you get involved in it again, it may be a long time before you see the light of day."[37] Similarly, in the county's second drug kingpin case, Dooley attributed profiteer motivations when sentencing Devon Johnson, another Black man: "Everyone has choices in life . . . but what you do in terms of selling heroin creates a lot of misery. . . . You're not using (drugs), you're not addicted, you're just selling to make money." For codefendant Maurice Rollins, the judge also drew on the image of a threatened community *and* nation: "Heroin is a scourge upon our community and the nation. . . . I hope you see where this is leading you."[38]

Anthony Guccia was one of three white defendants who pled guilty to felony third-degree criminal sale of a controlled substance and received a treatment-based alternative to incarceration. District Attorney Cornwell suggested that Guccia was dealing from a history of heroin addiction and not "just to make money." The judge agreed, noting that "anyone can be affected" by heroin, implying even a white community member. As he stated, "This is another disheartening tale of a person in this community whose life is destroyed by opiates. . . . This goes to show how heroin can affect anyone in this community. . . . There's only so many breaks you get. . . . You get this chance now and I hope you take advantage of it."[39]

Christopher Clerveau, a Black man, also pleaded to felony third-degree criminal sale of a controlled substance. Clerveau offered an alternative motive for dealing. It was not from addiction but financial hardship. A reporter described the courtroom interaction as follows:

> Clerveau . . . admitted he resorted to the criminal activity only when he found himself in dire financial straits and almost evicted. It's a choice,

he now says, that effectively ruined his life—he planned to get married this year.

"I made the worst mistake of my life," Clerveau said in court Wednesday, fighting back tears. "Within a moment of almost being evicted, I had to do the fastest thing I could do—I understand what I was doing was wrong."

Bounded by prearranged guidelines, Dooley sentenced Clerveau to eight years in prison. He recognized forty character letters sent to the court and confirmed his belief that Clerveau was not an "evil person." Yet, he reminded that dealing was "serious conduct," and he "could not overlook the role Clerveau played in catering to the community's share of the heroin epidemic." The judge added, "People grapple with financial problems. . . . Not everyone decides to sell drugs to make ends meet. . . . Selling drugs . . . is a crime that requires a lot of thought and is not generally a mistake someone makes in a split-second."[40] Certainly, sentencing involves a myriad of (albeit racially skewed) factors, including criminal record and possession amount.[41] Nevertheless, judge sentencing statements are cultural texts infused with racial meaning.[42] In this regard, judges dictate, in their sentencing, socially acceptable vocabularies of motive.[43] And, for Clerveau, economic circumstances that led him to deal did not suffice as proper motivation.[44]

Interviewee Aaliyah, a Black local organizer, observed a lack of media attention regarding financial motivations to deal: "It [the media] never discusses this fact that maybe this person's doing it because maybe he caught a felony charge, and he can't get a job. No one's hiring him, but he still needs to live and take care of himself. . . . 'This is what I know. This is why I'm doing this: easy cash, fast money.' But if you make it hard for a person to get a job out here, that's what they resort to. But then you're quick to hire 'em in prison and let them work for fifteen cents an hour." Michael, whom I cited previously, also offered several socioeconomic reasons why some people deal: "We mostly did it because we had to. We want food. We need to eat, and this is what we did. . . . The jobs wasn't there for us. Education was there, but who has time to be educated if your stomach is hungry?" Jim, a white user-dealer, further identified various reasons for his dealing: to use heroin, to support his family, and because he felt that the lifestyle was addictive in its own right.[45]

It should be said, furthermore, that the social conditions that drive some people to deal, such as poverty, marginalization, and organized abandonment, are not considered to be violent.[46] Rather, it is dealers who are deemed as violent.

Dealer-as-Violent: "A Fatal Drug Overdose Is Best in Their Business"

"Join us for the Buzz," a flier reads. The event is meant to provide conversation on "substance use prevention, addiction, recovery, and stigma." Visitors scatter throughout the public school theater. On the stage is an emergency medical technician (EMT) for the Tioga County Sheriff's Department.

He displays an image of fentanyl on the large projection screen behind him. "Just a few drops the size of salt can lead to a fatal overdose," he contends. "If I'm a drug dealer and cutting [fentanyl] with heroin, you would think I would be measuring very carefully how much, so I don't kill somebody. The answer is, 'No.' In their weird world, a fatal drug overdose is best in their business as all druggies want to know who has the hot stuff."

He warns, "As a responder or family member, if I'm going into my kid's room and fentanyl is there, I can easily overdose myself. There are numerous cases of law enforcement coming into physical contact with fentanyl who dermatologically overdosed and were revived."[47]

During the EMT's presentation, he drew on the dealer-as-violent trope, particularly when referencing dealers causing overdoses by maliciously cutting drugs with fentanyl and thereby putting (white) users, police, and the public at risk. In doing so, he offered two fearmongering myths that constitute the dealer-as-violent trope.

The first is that dealers cut drugs with fentanyl to create consumer demand.[48] Certainly, high-potency drugs can be appealing for some buyers, with news coverage even having an unintended advertising effect.[49] While there is an economic incentive to mix fentanyl with drugs, it is not due to the "weird world" of dealers but to the *weird world of drug prohibition*. Drug prohibition incentivizes dealers to transport compact substances, as was the case during alcohol prohibition.[50] It is simply cheaper for suppliers in Mexico, for instance, to produce and transfer synthetic drugs rather than to grow more labor-intensive, high-risk, and expensive opium.[51] And, on the street level, the dealer may not know what they are selling, and it is certainly not in their best interest to kill buyers. Drug sweeps, too, create a volatile market with unpredictable drug potencies. Interviewee Nate relayed that after Operation Get Money, buyers were seeking drugs from unknown online sources: "Everyone was panicking. People were tapping bags [cutting it with fentanyl], because they didn't have the real stuff anymore. . . . They had to get something to recoup, and they didn't know what else. So everybody started going to the black market [on the internet], getting fentanyl, and cutting it. Boom, everybody's dying . . . 'cause everything is gone. It was like a frantic running around trying to figure out what to do."[52] Such risk is compounded by a lack of access to fentanyl testing strips (which are used to detect fentanyl in substances) and safer consumption services.[53]

The second myth is that police are put at risk from fentanyl skin exposure. In 2016, the Drug Enforcement Agency (DEA) warned that a "very small amount" of fentanyl "ingested, or absorbed through your skin, can kill you."[54] Cases began to pop up. A police officer in East Liverpool, Ohio, claimed to have "[felt] his body shutting down" after brushing an unidentified white powder off his uniform after a routine traffic stop.[55] An officer in Harris County, Texas, felt "light-headed" from touching a flier someone put on her vehicle that was reported to have had the presence of fentanyl on it.[56] A New Hampshire man was charged with reckless conduct when, during a police visit, "some powder got on his index finger and [he] blew it off."[57] Despite such cases, it is a near scientific impossibility for overdose to occur from mere fentanyl skin contact.[58] Yet, these stories do much to bolster the image of police victimhood— and an attack on police is largely considered an attack on society itself.[59]

The dealer-as-violent trope also occurred in the Southern Tier when local reporters and lawmakers warned of drug-related gang violence. In "Gangs in the Tier," *The Press & Sun-Bulletin* connected instances of gun violence to gangs from New York City. The reporter stated, "A majority of gang members [the Bloods, Crips, Aryan Brotherhood, and Latin Kings] in the Broome County area hail from the New York City areas." In the same coverage, a nearby Elmira police chief expressed concern "about an ongoing turf war and the possibility that innocent bystanders might end up getting caught in the crossfire." The downstate Rockland County district attorney cited a "pipeline to death" where gangs and dealers prey on "a new generation of drug addicts . . . and often violently defend their 'turfs.'"[60] In response, New York Attorney General Eric Schneiderman created the Suburban and Upstate Response to the Growing Epidemic Initiative (SURGE) to, as a reporter stated, "target gangs and individuals who deal heroin and opioids, specifically in suburban and upstate communities."[61]

Despite such rhetoric and enforcement, gangs are not so well organized, and the randomness of gang-related violence, and street violence more generally, is overstated.[62] Dealer violence, too, is largely an outcome of drug prohibition. As licit markets rely on police violence to secure property, illicit markets too utilize a degree of violence, or a threat of violence, to address territorial and payment disputes.[63] Gangs can also provide a sense of belonging and protection within spaces of concentrated poverty and organized abandonment.[64] Interviewee Aaliyah spoke of community involvement by a local gang: "They did a lot. They were drug dealers, but they did a lot for the community, too. Every Christmas they had a big Christmas party, and they gave all the kids gifts. If you couldn't afford clothes for school, they would give sneakers. They would do shopping for the kids that needed clothes for school. They would do free haircuts, things like that. Because most of them had felonies, they couldn't get large jobs anyways. But they helped parents struggling. But, no, the media ain't talk about every time they had a Christmas party and was giving kids toys."

The dealer-as-violent trope consequently justifies police's own retaliatory violence. The justice scholar Bill Martin documented the Brome County and Binghamton police as having amassed a $275,000 armored personnel carrier, a South African Casspir, and "armored Humvees, large military trucks, night vision equipment and a wide assortment of military rifles."[65] Such weaponry makes for especially violent raids. Jim reflected on being raided by the Broome County Special Units Task Force:

> They knocked that shit [the door] down, marshals, special investigations unit. They come in like *Call of Duty*. [On the third and final raid, police retrieved seven bags of heroin.]

> Everybody's out there. It's fucking embarrassing, for seven bags. . . .
> You guys bust these people and make 'em out to be the biggest people in
> the world, Johnny Kingpin.

This practice is not just humiliating, but raiding police have killed pets, suspects, fellow police officers, and family and friends.[66] Indeed, they provide a haunting parallel with night raids during Reconstruction, in which white vigilantes—at times with police—terrorized, killed, and robbed Black people and their families.[67]

Yet, like economic conditions, police are not considered to be inherently violent. Rather, it is the monstrous dealer who is violent. And, as David Gilmore notes, "the horrible monster is always killed off, usually in the most gruesome manner imaginable by humans."[68]

Conclusion: "It Is Only a Matter of Time Before It Is Available Again"

The discourse of fear, as David Altheide notes, "promote[s] a sense of disorder and a belief that 'things are out of control.'"[69] Through the fear-generating dealer tropes, white communities become what Allen Feldman refers to as "paranoid space . . . where visible ordered spaces are subverted and intruded by unseen disordered spaces."[70] Police promise order by tracking and arresting the monstrous dealer to expel them from the social body.[71] "Get out or we will take you out," threatened the prosecutor's billboard, and the Sheriff's Office displayed mug-shot photos of those who were arrested on social media, with commenters referring to those presented as "scum," "trash," and "spreading that POISON in our towns." For bereaved parents, police and lawmakers promise retribution through dealer arrests and drug-homicide statutes. At a public forum I attended, the audience applauded when a white woman expressed gratitude to the police chief and sheriff, stating, "Every time you get dealers off the street, I thank you from the bottom of my heart."[72]

Yet, not only does policing bolster racist stereotypes and drug arrests, but it does not actually reduce the flow of illicit drugs.[73] Sergeant Matthew Cower of the Broome County Special Investigations Unit Task Force acknowledged as much when explaining why a 2018 $1 million seizure did not reduce drug sales, as evident with a subsequent 2022 takedown. He stated in reporting, "I wouldn't say we took so much of any drug off the street [in 2018 but] that it opened the market for another drug. . . . While we do seize a good amount of narcotics from the streets for our area, unfortunately it is still readily available. We might shut down a source of that drug to our area for a while; in my opinion, it is only a matter of time before it is available again." The same coverage cited Newtown Police Chief Tom Synan in Ohio as recognizing that drug busts even drive overdose rates: "It's more dangerous to have a disruption in the fentanyl supply because if that user doesn't have the fentanyl, the body's tolerances go down and when they go back to their normal doses, they have a higher chance of overdosing and dying because their body's not used to it." Even still, Synan recommended *expanding the role of police* to address the overdose rate, albeit through public health efforts: "We have to continue to do law enforcement . . . but we've got to expand our role to being links to the public health sector in getting those with chronic addiction into the health-care system so they can be treated."[74]

And so it continues: more policing for the supply and demand sides of the drug market. Indeed, that policing does not reduce drug use, dealing, or overdoses is essential for policing to continue, as police rely on fearmongering through an imagined monstrous Other. Police, as Travis Linnemann reminds us, "depend on the fear, terror, and horror of violence and crime for their own power."[75] And, as Cristina Rivera Garza puts it, "A society that is afraid is a society that looks down."[76] When it comes to drug supply and demand, there is not so much a concession of the failures of policing but, as Synan recommended, an incorporation of police as links to treatment. I cover such police-based treatment in chapter 3.

3

Caring Cops

Help with Handcuffs

In 2015, Gloucester, Massachusetts, Police Chief Leonard Campanello came to a realization, that in a time of rising opioid overdoses, people continued to be arrested "as much, if not more so," for possessing "an illegal, life ruining substance." He determined "a revolutionary new way to fight the war on drugs," in which "drug addicts [can] ask the police department for help." So, he established the Police Assisted Addiction Recovery Initiative, or PAARI (pronounced "parry"). Volunteers, referred to as "Angels," would receive calls from people seeking treatment, and they would "immediately be taken to a hospital and placed in a recovery program. No arrest. No jail." The organization's mantra speaks to a reimagining of narcotics policing: "Help instead of handcuffs."[1]

The following year, in 2016, the New York Joint Senate Task Force assured the state's commitment to police-based treatment initiatives, such as PAARI and Law Enforcement Assisted Diversion (LEAD). The task force promoted both programs when describing the overdose crisis as a public health issue: "Police departments statewide have adopted policies that reflect what Task Force contributors have repeatedly stated, 'This is a public health issue, we can't arrest our way out of the problem.' Programs such as Police Assisted Addiction and Recovery Initiative (PAARI) and the Law Enforcement Assisted Diversion (LEAD) connect drug users with necessary treatment rather than incarceration."[2] PAARI maintains forty-seven partners, which comprise police departments, county sheriff offices, and district attorney offices, and LEAD operates in twenty-three states and has seven sites in New York, including in the cities of Albany and Ithaca and in Dutchess, Niagara, Schenectady, and Schoharie Counties.[3]

While police treatment programs appear to be a reversal to law-and-order approaches to drug issues, policing does not merely operate through strict repression, but it does so through public health. Indeed, fifteenth-century police in Europe held administrative duties relating to "religion, health, morals, public safety, liberal arts, trade, [and] the poor."[4] While public health and police became separate institutions in the nineteenth century, public health initiatives continue to regulate the diseased and disordered subject. The Broome County Department of Health budget has suggested, for instance, that a comprehensive continuum of care for consumers would "provide for the *health and safety* of Broome County residents."[5] Police also show up in health-care settings, including in ambulances and emergency rooms, and they enforce public health mandates, for example, by arresting people for curfew violations from COVID-19 regulations.[6] To be sure, police are first responders for 911 calls, including for drug overdoses, as I document in the latter part of this chapter.

In the first two sections of this chapter, I explore police-based treatment in PAARI and LEAD in Broome County and Tompkins County, respectively. I identify what I refer to as *policing treatment*. Policing treatment occurs when officials announce treatment programming by rejecting traditional law-and-order approaches, declaring that "we can't arrest our way out of" an addiction crisis. Officials subsequently employ medical language to divide deserving "addicts" from undeserving dealers, and they deputize social workers and health-care providers to surveil participants. Program funding may also rely on drug-seizure money and the use of prospective program participants as confidential informants for dealer arrests. Moreover, through policing treatment, police are framed as benevolent, which, as Amanda Petersen puts it, "erases the *brutality and antagonisms* of racialized policing."[7] In turn, police maintain social order while appearing as caring cops.

PAARI: "We're Not the Enemy"

Broome County joined the PAARI initiative in 2015 through the Broome County Sheriff's Office Recovery Commitment (BCSORC). As the press release had it, Broome County municipal police departments would "serv[e] as eyes and ears on the ground and refer[] those suffering from the disease of addiction to the Sheriff's Office for placement in a treatment center." The Republican sheriff, David Harder, recognized the ubiquity of opioid addiction in the release, implicitly evoking an affected white community: "The opioid addiction epidemic has touched every community in the country, and here in Broome County, we are no different. As public servants, we have an obligation to help people in any way that we can. . . . By joining with PAARI, we can help people suffering from addictions reclaim their lives. These people are children, parents, cousins, friends, husbands, and wives, and we are tired of watching opioid addiction take them away from us." Port Dickinson Police Chief Douglas E. Pipher furthermore referred to opioid addiction as "a beatable disease" in the release: "People should not live in fear of their police departments. We are here to help, and when it comes to those suffering from addiction, we are going to prove it. . . . I have seen how it can make a real difference in people's lives and the lives of their family members and friends. Opioid addiction is a beatable disease."[8]

While these efforts laid the groundwork for the introduction of PAARI into Broome County, the most comprehensive initiative, which I take up in this section, was District Attorney Steve Cornwell's 2016 implementation of Operation S.A.F.E. (Save Addicts From Epidemic). Adopting Campanello's model, volunteers received calls and searched for out-of-state treatment beds, including in Pennsylvania, Florida, California, and Arizona. Cornwell confirmed in local reporting, "The addicts need to know they can reach out to law enforcement. . . . We're not the enemy."[9] Campanello praised the collaboration in a press release: "I am extremely proud to stand with Steve Cornwell and all of Broome County as we work together to fight the demand for heroin and other drugs in our community. He is a courageous leader."[10]

Interviewee Anna, a local mental health and drug policy advocate, expressed her initial excitement about the initiative: "I was so stunned to ever hear in my lifetime a district attorney wanting to set up a program to help people." Anna's enthusiasm was short-lived. She called to volunteer but did not receive a response: "I was all excited, and I never got called. . . . I'm on the volunteer list. I got my training. . . . We [interested volunteers] start talking to each other and found out none of us are being called." Interviewee Jane, a fellow advocate, felt that they had been dropped off the program for their community activism: "There were people that helped out with Operation S.A.F.E. in the beginning who are advocates and activists within the community, and somehow they got dropped off the program quietly. So people that really were showing out in the community, they really had a passion for that, that weren't brought into this program to be utilized." Anna's son, Simon, also did not receive a callback when reaching out for treatment. Anna continued, "[He] went to all those meetings with Operation S.A.F.E. with me, and even he got excited. When he was ready for help, . . . [he called]. . . . Nobody called him back." Simon was arrested a few days later and prosecuted by the same office. He felt "totally defeated," Anna reflected. "It's kind of like he [the DA] betrayed us. . . . Did you do it because you just got elected and you got all this press? . . . Okay, I get it, but there were people who were counting on it."

The program also restricted access for people who were incarcerated, who were on parole, who had a warrant out for their arrest, or who were on the sex offender registry. Interviewee Pamela contacted the DA on behalf of her son, Ryan, who had received a sex-offense conviction at nineteen years old and was incarcerated at the time of our interview. The office did not return his call, so Pamela pressed the DA:

> "Your son, there's no help for your son" is what he told me. And I said, "How can that be?"
>
> You know, he's still a person. Yes, he's done wrong, but there should be something for everybody. I don't care who you are.
>
> I said, "What do you want me to do, bury him?" And he said, "It's up to you, ma'am."

Given Ryan's difficulty in obtaining employment, treatment, and access to social services, Pamela concluded that the DA was right: There *was* no help for him. People with sex-offense records are, as Dale Spencer puts it of their bare life status, "physically in the community but rendered outside of it."[11]

The DA specified furthermore that the program was meant "to help local addicts" and not drug dealers.[12] Indeed, while funding came from donations and the national PAARI nonprofit, the initiative relied on traffic-diversion and drug-forfeiture funds.[13] Cornwell asserted in local reporting, "We can take the drug dealers' cars and cash and use it to help people struggling with addiction. . . . Let's make the drug dealers pay for the damage they have inflicted."[14] Two years later, he announced that police forfeited $281,572 from drug dealers and that approximately $70,000 went to state treatment and recovery services.[15] Further tying the program to drug arrests, the office also utilized participants as confidential informants, including for the county's largest drug seizure, Operation Get Money.[16] Interviewee Deborah, an advocate, informed, "They [people who use drugs] were actually working with the detectives. . . . They would—police would . . . [give them money] that they confiscated . . . to go out and buy drugs and get high but also to set people up."[17]

By dividing users from dealers, policing treatment operates through the ostensibly life-giving and death-generating dimensions of the carceral state. As Achille Mbembe puts it of necropolitics, "The ultimate expression of sovereignty largely resides in the power and capacity to dictate who is able to live and who must die." People are divided into a "sphere of common belonging against a sphere of others, or in other words, of friends and 'allies' and of enemies of civilization."[18] The death and domination of the dealer—as the enemy of civilization—is exemplified, both locally and more broadly, in arrest data, news coverage, forfeiture reports, mug shots, and police trophy shots of seized money, guns, and drugs.[19] With trophy shots, as Travis Linnemann puts it, police celebrate "everyday domination and death," as they hold down the arrested with gun in holster or hand.[20] Indeed, when not needed to appropriate Indigenous peoples' lands, the firearm, as Roxanne Dunbar-Ortiz reviews, "became a representation of ongoing racist domination—a kind of war trophy—not just of Native Peoples and their territories, but of African Americans and the world."[21]

Proof of death in Operation S.A.F.E. was coupled with proof of life for those who received treatment. The local newspaper published accounts of those who were sent to treatment, with one headline reading, "24 Addicts Up for Treatment."[22] The DA's office also confirmed in the county budget that the office had "placed an average of one addict a day into long-term treatment through Operation SAFE." In doing so, they reassured that the program "reduces crime and overdose deaths by getting addicts into treatment and off the street (where they commit crimes to pay for their addiction)."[23] Cornwell confirmed the life-generating outcome of the program in an emailed statement to a reporter: "The people we've sent to rehab are not out on the streets, stealing to feed their addiction, and their families and friends can finally rest at night knowing their loved ones are getting the help they need."[24] In policing treatment, police are deemed to afford life; they are angels, symbolized by the program logo of a halo over the letters "S.A.F.E."[25] But it is also a vengeful state. The DA announced when referring to the Operation Get Money arrests, "I make that offer to any of the buyers who are out there. . . . Maybe their drugs have dried up—instead of looking for another way, make the call now for treatment. If you end up selling drugs or possessing with the intent to sell, you will be charged."[26] With the thin blue line, as Linnemann reminds us, there are "only friends and foes, allies and adversaries, angels and demons."[27]

Even when accessing treatment, people who use drugs are subjected to police power, rendering life ever vulnerable. Consider the experience of interviewee Mark. His call was answered, and a treatment coordinator with the DA's office located a bed for him in California. Instead of the inpatient treatment Mark anticipated, he was set up in sober living and outpatient care with few resources.

> [Upon arrival], they're [the treatment providers were] like, "Um, so you got money for food, right?" And I'm like, "Um, no" [laughs].
> So, I'm going into this program with no clean time [he used heroin before leaving]. I'm out on the street. . . . And it happens to be a place where you can actually [get] methamphetamines [which] is actually my drug of choice.

He felt as though everything was "stacked against" him.

> Everything, everything was stacked against me. I didn't have money for copays for my meds, didn't have money for food. They got me this gift card. They went out of their way, but I was brought there [under] false pretenses big time.
> . . . My girlfriend had to send me a bus ticket [as he was unable to receive a plane ticket until completing the program].

Upon arriving back, Mark was arrested for a previous offense.

> Two days before I went there [to California], I got under arrest again. So I had all these pending charges stacked up against me, and they, just, they

issued a warrant when I was out there even though I came . . . through the DA's office. That doesn't really make sense [laughs].

. . . They knew if I got out there, they got their money, everybody got their money. . . . The DA knew I would just be a number for them.

For Mark, being a number, or "proof of life," was indicative of his fundamental disposability in the program.

These components of policing treatment—of police awakening narratives, program gatekeeping, and positive image work—also operate in Law Enforcement Assisted Diversion (LEAD).[28]

LEAD: "This Just Isn't Gonna Be for Us"

LEAD was founded in Seattle, Washington, in 2011. Police recommend program access for those who are arrested or who have a history of being arrested for low-level drug or prostitution offenses. Participants meet with a case manager for an evaluation and are offered housing, employment opportunities, treatment, and funds for food. An Operation Team, composed of a case manager, police officer, prosecutor, medical provider, and community representative, monitors participants. If they do not follow the guidelines set out by the team, the prosecutor may file charges. Initial evaluations found that LEAD reduced recidivism, criminal justice spending, and jail time; it increased housing, employment, and income/benefits access; and participants felt favorably toward the program.[29]

The promises of LEAD are highlighted in popular writing on the opioid crisis. In *Addiction Nation*, Anthony King describes LEAD as "restoring a sense of autonomy and control over one area of life," which allows people "to begin exercising control in more areas of their lives."[30] In *Unbroken Brain*, Maia Szalavitz refers to LEAD as "the rare law enforcement program based on harm reduction." As she explains, "The key idea is not to force people into abstinence and punish them if they fail, but rather, to connect them up with services that can help them meet their own goals—like finding a house or a job."[31] In downtown Seattle, she concludes, "LEAD officers are no longer the enemy."[32] Yet, like PAARI, there are aspects of policing treatment in LEAD, which were apparent in the initial development of LEAD in the city of Ithaca in the Southern Tier's Tompkins County.[33]

To address a rising rate of fatal overdose deaths in 2016, Ithaca Mayor Svante Myrick commissioned the "Ithaca Plan," a sixty-four-page report that included four pillars: prevention, treatment, harm reduction, and law enforcement. LEAD was part of the law enforcement pillar. It would "redirect law enforcement and community resources from criminalization to increasing access to services." The program would also "encourage a shared responsibility for community health and safety that extends beyond the Ithaca Police Department."[34]

The following year, a Community Police Board Meeting was held at City Hall. It was led by Ithaca Police Department (IPD) Officer Mary Orsaio and Sergeant Kevin Slattery. Officer Orsaio explained that the program was meant for nonviolent, low-level offenders "dealing with addiction": "As an officer, I have faced the same people over and over again for low-level offenses, and what I've found is that they're stuck in the system. . . . There has to be something else I can be helping (them) with besides putting cuffs on (them) and setting a court date." With LEAD, she detailed, case managers would work hand in hand with police "at a pace the client could keep up with." Orsaio added, "Small drug offenses will tie me up for a while between processing, fingerprinting and filing their criminal history. . . . That can sometimes take up to two officers. With small violations, if we can enroll them onto LEAD, it'll be quicker and get officers back on the road faster to do proactive work."[35]

Interviewee Dina, a white community organizer for a local jail reentry group, was originally optimistic about the program. Yet, she took issue with how LEAD was presented by police: "The police were . . . the ones who were like, 'We've seen this, how this doesn't work, and it's just cycling people in and out [of the criminal legal system].' . . . [It felt like they were saying,] 'Here's LEAD, here's how it works,' period. . . . And that was pretty much how it was coming out. . . . It felt like it stays with them because of the way it was presented to the public." Dina also expressed concern that police would focus on white people who use drugs, stating, "We're [police are] starting small so we have to start white, and then maybe we'll expand to Black people later." She met with a fellow organizer to document further concerns: There may be police bias in recommendations; recommendations without prior arrest might lead to actual arrests; prioritizing treatment beds for people in the program reduces broader treatment access; LEAD may function as a "snitch program"; and funding had been earmarked for a case manager but not for social services like housing, employment, or financial support.

Dina and other organizers called for an engagement meeting to, as she put it, "talk about . . . how we feel about it." She was emboldened by a LEAD Bureau presenter she met in New York's capital, Albany, who highlighted the importance of asserting community ownership over the program: "[The organizer told me,] 'Even if it says that the program isn't owned by any of these organizations, it certainly is not going to be owned by you unless you set it pretty forcefully,' so that is what we were doing." Word of the meeting was broadcast by the codirector of LEAD, which drew a police presence: "The codirector got word of it, and she sent out word to everybody who's involved. . . . Then the DA showed up, and the police showed up, legislators showed up. . . . Police [were] standing the whole time and delivering monologues about the program." The community stakeholder position was subsequently allocated to a group that, Dina felt, was less "in touch" with people coming out of the jail and less "boots on the ground." While remaining somewhat optimistic about the potential of LEAD, she resolved, "It's not going to be my thing."

Dina's experience is perhaps unsurprising. While the LEAD National Bureau designates the "community" as a stakeholder, the organization has highlighted police control over the program. The bureau has cited the importance of "officer and front line supervisor 'ownership'" and has recommended that police view the program as "business as usual," "just another tool," and not a "get out of jail free card."[36] The bureau has also reminded prosecutors that they hold discretion to file charges or not: "Whether they enter the program through an arrest diversion or a social contact referral, LEAD participants often have other pending cases that predate their LEAD entry or charges that are filed after they enter the program. . . . At every critical stage, there is an opportunity to use prosecutorial discretion in these cases to maximize the chances of a defendant changing their behavior." Prosecutors are also meant to "explain to case managers what clients need to do for the prosecutor to take favorable positions."[37] A case manager's remark on their role as a "good cop" in the original 2011 evaluation is telling of the relationship between service providers, police, and prosecution:

I like the way they play the bad cop and we get to be the good cop. And come and pick them up when they [police] have them in the alley. Or when they're getting picked up on the second arrest. And you get to make that decision, and the client knows that. The cops make them very aware of that—they're being the bad cop. But that also opens the door to build a better relationship with a client who's been less engaged in services and just kind of doing it their way. . . . So, yeah, I think it's good—took some ironing out, but it's a good relationship to maintain, definitely.[38]

LEAD adopts a community policing model, with one of the program's goals being to "strengthen the relationship between law enforcement and the community."[39] Yet, while community policing is meant to be "a collaboration between the police and the community that identifies and solves community problems," such practices tend to criminalize communities and enact intelligence gathering.[40] For LEAD, police set the boundaries of program access and community participation, and clients are framed as dangerous, or potentially dangerous, with another goal of LEAD being to "reorient government's response to *safety, disorder,* and health-related problems."[41] Community policing therefore operates as counterinsurgency, which, as David Correia and Tyler Wall put it, "relie[s] not simply on violence and destruction of enemy forces but also on implementing more friendly programs designed to gain the consent of policed populations."[42] Such programming, thus, "mask[s] occupation as cooperation."[43]

When thinking of the impetus for LEAD, I am reminded of Derrick Bell's "interest convergence." The concept refers to how racially progressive policies and legal decisions will more than likely maintain white elite dominance.[44] Indeed, LEAD was a compromise between the Washington State Public Defender Association's Racial Disparity Project and the Seattle Police Department (SPD). The former threatened litigation against the SPD for racial bias in arrest rates.[45] While LEAD has been shown to reduce racial disparities in arrests and provide services for marginalized participants, such programming nevertheless entrenches the police's role in service provision for housing, health care, job training, drug treatment, and mental health support. One Black community member spoke of LEAD this way: "This just isn't gonna be for us. You know what we call it? The criminal just-us system. No way we getting get out of jail free cards."[46]

Policing Overdose: "They Still Treated Me like I Was a Horrible Monster"

Policing public health does not solely involve treatment but occurs when police act as first responders for overdose revival. This is in spite of Good Samaritan laws that permit a person to call 911 to report an overdose "without fear of arrest" for possessing illicit substances or paraphernalia.[47] New York passed its Good Samaritan law in 2011, and by 2018, forty-five states had enacted such legislation.[48] In advocating for the law, the conservative Republican senator and Health Committee chair Kemp Hannon assured, "If someone is witnessing a drug or alcohol overdose, their first reaction should be to get help, not worrying about personal ramifications. This bill would alleviate some of the concern about charges an individual may face for illicit activity and provide quicker and more effective medical responses."[49] In our interview, the Broome County emergency medical services (EMS) coordinator spoke highly of the Good Samaritan law as a harm-reduction tool: "We've got the Good Samaritan law now, . . . and we're trying to just make it a little less risky, where we can—and it's that whole harm-reduction thing." Indeed, Good Samaritan laws have been shown to reduce opioid overdose deaths by 15 percent generally and by 26 percent for the Black non-Hispanic population.[50]

Nevertheless, as with policing treatment, Good Samaritan laws afford a number of policing mechanisms—namely, selectivity for who is protected and the ongoing criminalization of callers and those who are revived. In this, Good Samaritan laws maintain practices of *policing overdose*, which refers to the ways in which overdose revival is policed, both in one's ability to seek revival and in the circumstances in which revival occurs.

Indeed, not all callers are protected from arrest. A flier published by the New York Department of Health (DOH), "New York State's 911 Good Samaritan Law Protects YOU," affords a visual depiction of the criteria. In the right column, it informs that callers are protected for possessing controlled substances including A2 felony offenses (anything under eight ounces), possessing alcohol where underage drinking is involved, possessing any quantity of marijuana, possessing drug paraphernalia, and sharing drugs. The left column lists those who are not protected, including for an A1 felony possession of a controlled substance (eight ounces or more), for selling or intending to sell controlled substances, for having open arrest warrants, and for probation or parole violations.[51] These criteria omit a number of people who use drugs, particularly those who are involved with the criminal legal system. As Black and Latinx people are disproportionately criminal justice involved, they are, as a whole, less protected from further arrests. Even while these laws have reduced fatal overdose rates, they still bolster a racially divided policing system and thus contribute to, as Ruth Wilson Gilmore defines of racism, "the state-sanctioned or extralegal production and exploitation of group-differentiated vulnerability to premature death."[52]

Further factors put callers at risk. Undocumented immigrants risk deportation.[53] Parents risk Child Protective Services (CPS) removing their children. Tenants and Section 8 housing residents risk eviction. Employees risk being fired. Sex workers risk arrest, while facing an increased likelihood of police violence if they are gender diverse.[54] The caller also risks homicide charges if the person does not recover from the overdose. Drug Policy Alliance (DPA) attorney Lindsay LaSalle makes this point well: "People are not going to call 911. . . . The increased prosecution of drug-induced homicide completely undermines those laws."[55]

Speaking to such risk, interviewee Kay mentioned a case in which a woman dropped her overdosing friend on the side of the road, presumably for fear of calling the police: "I have this friend, who was also my ex, who was dropped on the side of the road two blocks from Wilson Hospital. [He was] pulled out of a car in the middle of winter when he was overdosing and left to die. . . . Because they didn't call. They were too scared to take him to the hospital. They were afraid, because you are treated differently even if you call with something like that. He was ready to be sober." She had mixed feelings about the driver, as she recognized the situation she was in as a person who uses drugs:

But a lot of these dealers are addicts themselves, and, I mean, I used to be so angry with the girl that my best friend was with when it happened. I mean, I was so angry with the fact she just pulled him out of the car and left him there to die. I'll never forgive her for that, but at the same time, she's an addict herself. She was doing what she knew. I can be angry and pissed off at her, but I also have to be compassionate, too, because who knows what she had on her. Even if she called, she probably would have been arrested for driving. She probably would have been arrested for whatever she had on her.

Indeed, Kay was harassed by police when she called to report an overdose, despite being sober at the time: "If you're an addict, and you've been through it, and you call to help somebody else, you get treated like shit. . . . I was thrown up against a car, and I was the one that called, and I was sober. I had had two years sober, and they still treated me like I was a horrible monster."

Not just the caller but the overdosed person can also be subjected to police violence. The revived have been described by officers as angry and violent.[56] Certainly, after an overdose, one can be in a state of panic, confusion, and agitation—compounded by police interaction.[57] Yet, such an impression of the overdosed readies police for violent intervention that appears as a kind of knee-jerk reaction. Hope Smiley-McDonald and colleagues interviewed police officers and quote one officer describing their use of violent force after the revived "grab[ed] a medic": "I have had a few people get legitimately upset with you because you ruined their high. I try to stay close because some people do come out swinging. I had one grab a medic and I had to kick them in the face."[58] When police responded to an overdose call in a Rite-Aid parking lot in Philadelphia, as Philip Kavanaugh further reports, "the revived man began vocalizing unintelligibly and 'striking parked cars and the ground with his body.'" In response, an officer punched him in the head "with a closed fist" as "other police attempted to handcuff him."[59] Even when people are compliant, the threat of force remains. An interviewee in Smiley-McDonald and colleagues' sample stated that, once a person is revived, "you can go to the hospital without handcuffs or with handcuffs, you decide."[60] Indeed, Wisconsin police have recommended handcuffing overdosed people.[61] In this regard, police are always poised for violence, even for people who are on the verge of death.[62]

Police contact can also lead to questioning, search, and humiliation. Interviewee Lisa spoke about her experience of being revived, questioned, left at the hospital, and returning to a torn-apart car:

I was just dead two minutes ago, and now I'm fucked up—you know I am—and now you're asking me shit. . . . "Where's your needles? Where's your shit? Where'd you get it?"

. . . What I ended up doing is, I gave him my empty bags. . . . And like my thought was, "Okay, what if there is something in it?" Which I know is not the case, but then he's like, "Well, you could save someone else's life," and stuff like that. So I gave him whatever I had, and he actually, when I went back, I guess they tore my car apart.

. . . I don't remember if I said, "Yeah, go ahead." . . . Actually I'm thinking back, I might have just said, "It's in the glove box." I don't know, but what happened is they left everything right there. Like, I went back to get my car, and there was needles all over the ground. . . . There's bags, there's everything.

. . . And when I got to the hospital, it was awful. Like, you're strapped to the gurney. They bring you into the waiting room in this fuckin' gurney. They literally just dropped me, and they're like, "Okay, have a nice day."

As a final note, police also monitor harm-reduction providers, such as syringe-service programs that offer clients syringe-exchange IDs meant to protect them from being charged for possessing a new or used syringe. Interviewee Gabi, who worked in a local program, discussed police surveillance of their location: "Sometimes police will just sit outside of our building. . . . They know who's going to be coming and going, and they just sit there. I don't really know any arrests directly from that, but it definitely makes our clients really nervous." Interviewee Sarah received a possession charge, despite having a card from a local exchange:

So I caught four hypodermic charges. I had a [syringe-service program] card, and . . . three of the times I didn't have it on me. The one time I did have it on me, I had a clean needle, didn't even use it. It was brand new. I had it in my boot. I had my [program name] card in my pocket, and the police would not take my [program name] card. They would not accept it. They still charged me with it. They said, "That's not acceptable. We don't care," pretty much. And the other . . . three times, . . . I said, "Call [program name] because I do have a [program name] card. You're supposed to call to verify." . . . They were like, "We're not wasting our time doing that."

Police have also taken to raiding syringe-service offices, as Travis Lupick documents in *Light Up the Night*.[63] Within racial capitalism, no one, to be sure, is outside the scope of policing.

Conclusion: Policing Treatment as State Violence

A small-town police chief who is himself in long-term recovery speaks to a packed crowd in Albany. It is a recovery event hosted by statewide advocates. He tells of the merits of PAARI, to which the crowd offers thunderous applause:

"I requested the police department attempt police-assisted recovery, and the Lieutenant said, 'jump,' and we jumped. . . . The first person who showed was embraced with hugs. In eight months, seventy-eight people had been helped, all from six different counties, and not one person was turned away. I get to talk about seventy-eight miracles that occurred. We do whatever is necessary for any person who is walking this earth to come in and say, 'I have a medical condition. Please help me.' It is proof that you do not need a lot of money or time. If you have the will, anything can happen."[64]

While certainly many state actors are sincere in their desire to help people who use drugs, such rhetoric does more to bolster police's public legitimacy by framing them as benevolent caregivers. Police's use of Narcan, for instance, as Kavanaugh contends, "functions as a symbol, reminding citizens and communities that police are not some violent inimical force," and it "emphasizes their beneficent duty to protect, serve, and save."[65] Actions by individual officers and departments, too, presume a "good apple" theory of policing, in which caring officers ripen the bunch. Yet, *violence* is, as Micol Seigel reminds us, "fundamental to police."[66] Policing treatment, in turn, is *help with handcuffs*, if not for the person who seeks treatment, then for the dealer—and both are always subject to state violence.[67] A similar form of treatment-based carceral violence is evident in drug treatment court.

4

Caring Courts

A Controlling Embrace

On April 24, 2017, Southern Tier resident Jennifer Grenchus tragically ran her car into the forty-seven-year-old pedestrian Ronald Richardson. She dragged him 120 feet before stopping. "It's horrific; nobody should see this," a witness told a reporter.[1] Grenchus was charged with vehicular manslaughter and pled to the lesser offense of criminally negligent homicide. Her attorney argued for leniency, as she was battling cancer treatments and addiction; she had morphine and fentanyl in her system at the time of the crash. "Close monitoring . . . would ensure she stays on the right path," her attorney assured. Broome County Court Judge Kevin Dooley agreed and sentenced her to five years of probation with time served, as she had spent eleven months in jail. He warned, "Addicts ruin their own lives, they ruin the lives of their family. . . . In this case, you took the life of another person, so I'm going to keep a close eye on you. . . . The time has come for you to overcome addiction. . . . You should do it for your daughter, you should do it for your family." Grenchus responded in kind, "I did make a horrible decision. I took an innocent life. Because of the remorse I feel, I've been forced to question who I am. . . . I'm truly sorry for what I've done."[2]

Akin to the white resident Anthony Guccia, discussed in chapter 2, Grenchus was viewed by the judge in a sympathetic manner. She was encouraged to "overcome addiction" to be a good mother for her daughter.[3] Yet, she was not off the hook entirely. The judge would keep a "close eye" on her, expressing the gendered paternalism of the state.[4] After eleven months in jail, she was sentenced to probation, in which she would be required to meet with a probation officer and be subjected to unannounced home visits.[5] Like policing treatment, treatment-based probation is nevertheless justified through the medical framing of addiction as a disease. After all, probation was meant for Grenchus "to overcome addiction."[6] This dynamic is perhaps no more evident than in drug treatment court.

Originally implemented in 1989 in Miami, Florida, drug court programming utilizes a carrot-and-stick approach to addiction recovery.[7] Broadly speaking, access is afforded to those who are charged with a drug-related nonviolent crime. Participants work with a drug court team made up of criminal justice officials and treatment providers. Judges offer awards for program success, including gift cards, lessened restrictions, and progression through program phases. They simultaneously allocate sanctions for program violations, including essay writing, community service, and jail time. If participants are terminated from the program, the original charges stand. If they are successful, charges are reduced or dropped. As Sam Quinones puts it in *The Least of Us*, "With prison hanging over [participants]," drug courts have "a chance to pry them from dope's mastery and toward recovery."[8] Or, as drug court advocates have put it simply, "It works!"

While drug courts have a decades-long history, the opioid crisis has breathed new life into court-based treatment. Drug courts have been supported by the Obama, Trump, and Biden administrations, including in the 2022 Safer America Plan.[9] There are over four thousand drug treatment courts in the US.[10] As of 2016, New York hosted 124 drug courts, and there is a growing number of opioid courts, such as the Buffalo Opioid Intervention Court and the Bronx Opioid Avoidance and Recovery Court.[11] Over ninety-three thousand people have participated in a New York State drug court program.[12] Established in 2002, the Binghamton Adult Drug Treatment Court was also meant to play a role in addressing the opioid crisis. In 2017, the Broome County district attorney promoted drug courts in the "Safer Streets. Brighter Future" initiative, along with police treatment diversion. The office informed the county of the program's success: "For those charged with a crime, we have increased the number of cases diverted to drug court which will prevent future crimes by helping addicts address their addiction issues and avoid jail and a criminal record."[13] In what ways do drug courts frame addiction, treatment, and criminal justice?

In this chapter, I explore drug court surveillance and addiction identity construction in the Binghamton drug court. First, I outline more generally how drug courts operate through what Dawn Moore refers to as "therapeutic surveillance," which blends care and control through overlapping disciplinary regimes, ostensibly for participants' well-being.[14] I then hone in on how therapeutic surveillance is made sensible through the in-court construction of a drug court participant addiction identity, as I observed in open court sessions.[15] This identity deems participants as both "criminal addicts," associated with racialized disorder, and "recovering addicts," associated with white civil order. Participants must navigate, negotiate, and, ultimately, perform this bifurcated identity for program success. Finally, I consider interviewees' experiences with the local drug court, particularly regarding surveillance, service access, and its reliance on incarceration. From this, I contend that, as with policing treatment, drug court programming, through a disease framework of addiction, entrenches the criminal legal system within addiction recovery, while presenting the image of caring courts.

Surveilling the Criminal Addict: The Team Is Watching

In outlining therapeutic surveillance, Moore adopts Michel Foucault's conceptualization of "pastoralism," which "is an individualized form of power which relies on the vigilance of the shepherd to lead his flock to salvation. In this sense, pastoral power is always essentially benevolent, temporary, transitional and, above all, watchful."[16] Unlike the shepherd, however, therapeutic surveillance operates through "a range of actors" who "contribute to monitoring each individual participant."[17] In drug court, this includes a coordinator, defense attorney, district attorney, judge, probation officer, and treatment provider. The group observes participants in their daily lives, at home, in school, and at work. Participants share with the court their "feelings, thoughts, attitudes, and beliefs" and watch each other for mutual accountability.[18] As such, therapeutic surveillance, as Moore reminds us, "is neither technocentric nor dystopic but rather intimate, pastoral and productive."[19] In this section, I consider the various sites of surveillance that drug courts operate through—inside and outside the courtroom.

Drug courts restrict participants from going to places and interacting with people deemed to trigger drug use; courts, thus, carve out chunks of socio-spatial life into healthy and unhealthy zones.[20] The local drug court, for instance, restricts housing, contact with people on probation or parole, and visiting establishments where alcohol is served. This put Kimberly in a bind, as she relayed to the judge in open court. As she told it, after a mandated Alcoholics Anonymous meeting, she was unable to patronize a bowling alley with members because it served alcohol. Participants can also be surveilled through electronic monitoring.[21] Julian was placed on an e-monitoring device for a probation violation. He was on house restriction at the area residential reentry center, or "halfway house." He violated his restriction, and in open court, the team warned him that they may mandate him to an inpatient residential treatment center. E-monitoring devices, therefore, as James Kilgore puts it, have the capacity not only to "control movement and behavior but to convert human activity into data and use that data to punish (or in rare instances, reward) the wearer."[22]

As evident in Julian's case, drug courts at times require participants to attend inpatient treatment. Inpatient centers largely follow the Hazelden model of community support, which relies on twelve-step programming and operates through the idea that someone needs to hit rock bottom before recovering.[23] Samaritan Daytop Village, an inpatient center that has worked with the Binghamton drug court, describes such an approach in marketing material: "Our treatment programs provide intensive, highly structured treatment environments using the principles of the therapeutic community model as their foundation."[24] Yet, critics have pointed out that inpatient approaches tend to involve group shaming, forced abstinence, nonconfidential counseling, and drug testing, and staff often hold pessimistic views of clients.[25] Inpatient treatment programs thus run on, as Maya Schenwar and Victoria Law argue, "prison-like principles," as "they confine people under strict watch, hold them to a fixed schedule, and regulate their movements and what they do with their bodies."[26] Interviewee Rebecca stated of a local drug and alcohol program that worked with the court, "They're very strict, and they—like, the first month in there, they [clients] can't go outside. They can't leave. And it's called . . . a 'blackout.'" If clients "get in trouble," they are required to submit to "personal reflection time." "It's basically like you're grounded," she added.

Drug courts also mandate outpatient treatment, in which participants are drug tested and required to participate in nonconfidential counseling. Drug testing comprises what Nancy Campbell refers to as "technologies of suspicion," as they act as "technological forms of supervision, monitoring, supposed deterrence, and ultimately control."[27] Such testing is stigmatizing and humiliating and can lead to jail incarceration. Interviewee Gabi, who worked for a local harm-reduction provider and sat on the drug court panel, discussed her concern regarding the team's use of stigmatizing language and reliance on jail incarceration from drug testing: "When someone came up positive [for a drug test], not only do they not use terms like 'came up positive,' they still say, 'gave a dirty,' you know what I mean? But their solution was to remand them to the county jail. I think enough evidence has been shown that that's not safe, so still using those antiquated practices is kind of just dangerous." Drug court participants are also required to meet with a counselor. Sadie Ryanne Baker, a transwoman and mental health activist, has stated that coerced counseling fuels "the client's sense of powerlessness, which is one of the primary causes and consequences of trauma."[28] Indeed, as information is sent to the court, it can lead to sanctions, including jail time.

Drug court participants must also fulfill a variety of social obligations: They are required to maintain or seek employment, complete community service hours, and attend sober support meetings, which are most often twelve-step in orientation.[29] Supervisors, meeting chairs, and treatment providers track their attendance. On top of this, they must report to the drug court regularly. Gabi reflected on the expectations placed on participants: "Some people have two times a day reporting [to the drug court], and that's a lot, to live wherever you live at, report twice a day downtown to drug court to test, still make it to groups, still navigate DSS [Department of Social Services], and appointments. It's a lot." In moving from monitored treatment to community service to employment to drug testing to counseling to social service providers, participants are placed on, to borrow from Emma Russell and colleagues, a *treatable* carceral churn, which refers to the production of *treatable* carceral subjects via the disciplined movement of people through the *therapeutic* carceral circuits.[30] And, if participants complained in the local court, the judge appealed to their individual tenacity—that when they wanted to get drugs, "they would move mountains," but they "have barriers in the mind to go to recovery and treatment." As the city's website states of drug court success, *"Attitude is Everything."*[31]

Finally, drug court participants are surveilled directly in the courtroom. Before sessions, the Broome County case coordinator randomly handed out oral drug-testing sticks, bailiffs walked around the courtroom, and the judge monitored eye rolls and side conversations. During one session, he sent two women participants from the public courtroom benches to the jury box for talking during check-ins. The judge also reminded of his watchful eye outside the courtroom. He stated to Angela, who had missed appointments and claimed that she had been sick, that he saw her "in the sun yesterday," thus diminishing her excuse. When Carey discussed moving residences, the judge teased that he "now can't drive past and check" in on her. In another humorous exchange, David relayed that in a dream, he was eating tacos on a Saturday night, and in the same dream, the judge asked if he "should be doing that." David joked that the judge must have "wanted to make sure he was doing the right thing." Interviewee Sarah took a more serious tone regarding the drug court team: "They watch you. They follow you."

How is therapeutic surveillance in drug court programming—as based on the regulation of movement, drug testing, and coerced counseling—made sensible for addiction recovery? In the following section, I observe how participants are made to adopt a drug court addiction identity as "criminal addicts" and "recovering addicts." In tracking addiction identity formation, I locate a drug court narrative habitus, or typical way of doing things in the courtroom, which organizes power, surveillance, and subject formation.[32] To borrow from Summerson Carr in *Scripting Addiction*, the courtroom acts as a *normalizing site*, "where people learn to represent themselves in a manner that supports existing institutional and cultural orders."[33] And, certainly, a drug court participant's ability to represent themselves through ritual performance "has far-reaching material and symbolic consequences."[34] Participants are thus *storied* into drug court programming as objects of care and control in the stage drama of the courtroom.[35]

Creating Criminal Addiction in Drug Court

In the following, I examine how the drug court identity is constructed in typical open court sessions in the Binghamton drug court. Identity construction occurs when participants sign the court contract, receive awards and sanctions, and are terminated or graduate from the program.

Signing the Contract

Morning sessions begin at 9:00 a.m. Participants stand in front of the judge with the defense attorney and prosecutor at their side. Given pretrial incarceration, many are outfitted in a county-issued orange jumpsuit. The judge reads rights lost when signing, which include a swift and determinant sentence, to remain silent, to confidentiality with attorney and treatment specialists, to protections against unreasonable search and seizure (for drug screening), and to certain rights to appeal.[36] He verifies that they signed freely, spoke with an attorney, and were able to read and comprehend the contract. He also confirms that "no substance interfered with the ability to understand the contract." Once signed, the document is entered into the court record.

The judge inquires about the defendant's charge or charges, reminding them that they have lost the right to remain silent. At this point, participants are made to associate their criminal offense to their drug addiction through storied exchange. After all, drug court is, as the handbook has it, "designed for people who have *criminal charges* and an *addiction* to drugs/alcohol."[37] Standing in front of the judge, Dan admitted to stealing property from his employer. The judge clarified, "You sold for addiction?" Dan confirmed, "Yes." Susan was charged with endangering the welfare of a child when overdosing on heroin in a parked car with her son. The judge encouraged Susan, "That you overdosed with a child should be motivation to make changes." These stories thus act as court-based rock-bottom moments, as they feature "a downward spiral of substance abuse, the reaching of a crisis point which is the catalyst for epiphany, then the upward climb of recovery."[38]

The judge presumes subsequent recovery through drug court participation. He stated to Madison, "The program is a chance to have hopes and dreams again, to get rid of the shackles, not only of jail but of addiction, . . . to get the life you are entitled to." If participants do not take this opportunity, he warns that their criminal-addict lifestyle will lead to prison or death. As he told Robert, "It's about change, right? It's about change and opportunity, but you need to change. Otherwise, it is a vicious cycle of jumpsuit and chains. If you do not work with the program, you will end up in prison or dead. You want to live, right?" During this exchange, carceral imagery of the jail, jumpsuit, and chains symbolizes participants' current carceral status as "criminal addicts"—and potential hopes and dreams through productive citizenship.

While the drug court signing is a formal part of the plea agreement, the exchange is telling: It is where a bifurcated drug court addiction identity is established through storied interaction.[39] First is the current "criminal addict" identity, evident by the defendant's addiction-related criminal behavior. Their admission is key, as the handbook states, "drug court is for people who *admit* they have a problem with drugs/alcohol."[40] It is, in turn, an assertion of their own powerlessness *and* willingness to submit to the court. With this, the judge promises that the participant has the opportunity to "have hopes and dreams again" as a productive citizen. The caring and controlling hands of the court are meant to be *life-generating*; but, if the participant does not take the opportunity, the state is also *death-generating*, as their criminal-addict lifestyle will presumably lead to imprisonment or death.[41]

Subsequently, in the afternoon sessions, participants are made to demonstrate their adoption of the "recovering addict" identity against the always looming "criminal addict" identity. This occurs when they receive awards and sanctions.

Caring for the "Recovering Addict": The Carrot Approach

Progress meetings are held every Tuesday from 2:45 to 4:00 p.m. Each participant stands in front of the judge, with onlookers remaining on the public courtroom benches. The judge confirms drug test results, reads treatment/probation reports, reviews progress goals, and asks, "What is an important thing you did for recovery since you were last seen?" Participants provide updates on employment, education, meeting attendance, gaining a sober support network, finding hobbies, living independently, finishing mandated community service hours, and maintaining proper diet and exercise.

Once updated, the judge ties participants' accomplishments to the "right living" that productive citizenship affords, which is based on emotional regulation, health, law-abiding behavior, sobriety, time management, and a strong work ethic.[42] He praised Samantha for using a planner to become more organized. Jane received applause for passing her road test after two years of driving without a license, and Bob assured that his anger-management classes improved his communication skills. The judge provided support and recognized personal development for Skyler, who had been facing family difficulties, for "staying strong": "This would have destroyed you before, but you are staying strong and progressing."

Participants receive further praise when transitioning between the three program phases. To progress, they are required to tie their "life story" to ongoing drug court success. When moving to phase 2, the judge stated for Tarek, one of the few Black participants, "I want to hear your life story, want to know your experiences, what journey led to drug court. That helps us [the drug court team] know what you've gone through and how we can help you. This is identified with your last incident [the arrest], [as] old behavior can lead down the wrong path." As such, participants are meant to go "gut level," as Allison McKim puts it, by tying their past trauma and present struggles within the context of drug court recovery.[43] The carceral churn, in this sense, is an emotional one, as participants are made to dig deep in mandated support groups, in counseling, to the drug court team, and in open court. The latter, too, proffers state-sanctioned voyeurism, where onlookers—myself included—can witness medical, familial, and emotional aspects of participants' lives.[44]

When transitioning phases, participants are asked to "say a few words" to the audience, in turn acting as institutional role models.[45] Facing onlookers, and becoming more audible, Allie recommended that they stick with the program—as it afforded her a "new life." Roger remarked, "When I first started, I had a chip on my shoulder. I did not want to deal and thought I could just not use and float through. I had to start listening to these guys, and it's working." While those who are transitioning are told to "speak from the heart," their statements are shaped by a drug court narrative habitus: They are expected to accept individual responsibility, recognize their personal transformation by "surrendering to the court" (with some adding God or their Higher Power), and express positive change through productive citizenship. The judge subsequently frames drug court as the catalyst for their recovery, entwining participants' life stories with the life-generating power of the program.

As with signing the contract, progress meetings are key for drug court addiction identity formation, as participants are made to link their progress within an overarching recovery narrative grounded on productive citizenship. While awards speak to the participant's "recovering addict" identity, sanctions ensure that their simultaneously court-constructed "criminal addict" identity is kept in check.

Controlling the "Criminal Addict": The Stick Approach

The judge allocates sanctions for noncompliance. Noncompliance includes showing up late to court, missing meetings, failing drug tests, receiving negative reports by treatment providers and probation officers, and engaging in "disruptive or disrespectful behavior" in the courtroom.[46] Slip-ups are to be expected. Yet, noncompliance is viewed by the court as leading to a downward spiral into an "old" criminal drug lifestyle.[47] Such behaviors are "triggers" that send participants, as the judge would put it, "down a path that would lead to relapse" and, eventually, prison or death. The judge responded to Matt's failure to look for sober support by asserting, "You can't cut corners. You have to give 100 percent. What will you do? Go back to jail? No, you're gonna die. You need to wake up that this is life and death. For recovery . . . you need to figure out what's going wrong as self-examination. . . . I'm willing to work with each individual . . . for a plan that works for you. I want to save your life."

Sanctions, such as essay writing, added community service hours, and even jail time, are deemed necessary to put the participant back on track. The judge required Diana, who had been arriving late to court and mandatory meetings, to write an essay on the importance of being on time. James was reprimanded with a weekend of community service for showing up late for drug testing and missing outpatient meetings. Mark was mandated to spend a weekend in jail for driving without a license. Indeed, participants are at times handcuffed and led out of the room as a show of therapeutic force.[48] The judge affirmed that those sent to jail were an "example" for others: "If I feel you are making an effort and taking action into your own hands, I don't think there is a need for jail. When you are not and cutting corners, then that's when I get pissed off, and that's when I send people to jail as an example."

Sanctions, to reiterate, are not meant merely to punish but to support recovery.[49] The judge reminded Audrey that jail incarceration was to stress the importance of being honest, as dishonesty is a trigger that leads to relapse. For Steven, who was mandated to jail for the weekend, it was his "dishonesty" about driving a car without a license that he needed to reflect on. The judge instructed, "When you are there, think about honesty and actions consistent with recovery." When participants complete sanctions, they are expected to communicate positive self-transformation, that the punishment was a "learning experience."[50] When Tom was asked what he gained from added community service hours, he stated that he "enjoys helping the community." The judge pressed further, "Think of why." Tom responded, "It helps me slow down." This appeared satisfactory, as "slowing down" communicated improved emotional restraint as part of a newly transformed self.

If a participant explains their noncompliant behavior outside of individual accountability, they are viewed as being in denial, playing the victim, not having an incentive to change, or making excuses and rationalizations.[51] They are not, as the judge would contend, "being honest" with themselves or the court, which is a clear sign of so-called criminal-addict behavior. When missing mandatory support meetings, Angela, whom I documented in the previous section, informed that she was sick and had a medical note to prove it. The judge relayed that he saw Angela outside the previous day and that if she let distractions interfere with her recovery, she would be "down the road to relapse." That is why, he continued, meetings are so important. Angela was caught between a bifurcated narrative identity, where she could either accept the sanction (revealing her "new" "recovering addict," productive-citizen identity) or reject it (revealing her "old" "criminal addict" identity).[52] She accepted the judge's interpretation and, once facing the audience, rolled her eyes and whispered a negative retort—thus enacting a small moment of narrative defiance.[53]

The imposed dueling identities of "recovering addict" and "criminal addict" are realized at the end of the program, when participants are terminated or graduate.

Graduation and Termination

Those who regularly violate or do not portray positive development are at risk of being terminated from the program. When this occurs, participants have the opportunity to present to the judge in morning sessions. Miles, a Black participant, admitted his infraction and assured his progress by distancing from his "old self." He confirmed, "I appreciate drug court. . . . I am more clear and have a better idea of recovery, recovery from old behaviors and old self." Barb was terminated for not demonstrating personal transformation. She was, the judge relayed, "unwilling to change." She had the best opportunity to "break the cycle" but "threw it out the window." He asserted, "I have seen you go downhill, and each time I see that it gets worse. You are not ready to change things or be honest."

Justin was terminated for absconding for a year. The judge declared, "It is a sad day." Justin, in shackles and jumpsuit, remained silent. The judge pushed, "You don't think so? Let me tell you, I've been working in criminal justice for thirty-one years. When I tell you it's a sad day, it's a sad day." He forecasted Justin's future: "You're going to prison. You'll get out and use again." Justin interjected that he had not used drugs during the period he absconded. The judge retorted that it was "not just about using" and that Justin had "used [up] his time to speak." He confirmed that Justin had not taken the opportunity provided by drug court and ended up "in cuffs and chains." Further treatment would not suffice. The judge added, "From your attitude, you are a real criminal. You are not doing it from addiction." He directed the bailiff, "All set. Please take him away."

In contrast, those who graduate are celebrated in a local theater attended by public officials, the drug court team, reporters, fellow participants, and friends and family. Graduates speak onstage, narrating positive transformation from program completion—that "today, life is beautiful," as the graduate Chris confirmed. They recall early childhood experiences (positive and negative), a downward spiral that led them to drug court, initial resistance to and assumptions about the program (thinking it was a "get out of jail free card"), surrendering to the court, and eventual success—gaining a sober life and enjoying new or secured jobs, educational achievements, and familial bonds. As Tracy stated at the podium, "Drug court saved my life, and I will always be grateful."

In termination and graduation, the final addiction identity of the participant is realized. One is of a "criminal addict" who is "unwilling to make changes" or, as in Justin's case, is a "real criminal" who is "not doing it from addiction." They are marked for disposability through prison or death. For those who graduate, they await a new life grounded in productive citizenship as a "recovering addict." The success of drug court—and its mechanisms of care and control—is therefore measured through graduates' narrated transformation from an "old" "criminal addict" self into a "new" productive-citizen self. As the DA affirmed onstage when speaking to graduate success, "The takeaway is treatment can work. Recovery is possible, so spread the word. It is proof right here." The life-generating and death-generating dimensions of the court— borne on the bifurcated drug court addiction identity—is thus realized.

Does It Work?

I was speaking with Megan at a local coffee shop about her drug court experience. She felt, like those who presented at graduation, that drug court "can save your life." "I've been on drug court for like fifteen months. . . . Thank God I was in drug court because it, you know, it kept me structured, and it kept me on the right path. . . . It can save your life, you know, because they truly, genuinely care. They're not just trying to get you through the program. They're going to keep you until they feel as though you're ready, so I'm just super grateful that I got a chance to, one, get rid of my charges, but [also] to get my life back together." Megan proclaimed a positive experience, a point stated not only in the courtroom and on the graduation stage but also in a confidential setting. Nevertheless, the success of drug court is questionable. Drug court graduation rates range from 30 to 70 percent.[54] In New York, 93,000 people had participated in drug court by the end of January 2020. Of these, 42,800 graduated, meaning that 50,200, or 53 percent, were terminated.[55] And, those who were terminated were likely to receive longer sentences than if they had not participated at all.

Interviewee Sarah was terminated from drug court. While in the program, she broke her back and was prescribed pain medication. The court coordinator told her, as Sarah recalled, "You can't take opiates. You're a drug addict, blah, blah, blah." Sarah continued to take her prescription, which was not enough, as she had indeed been using opioids, unbeknownst to the court. She missed meetings and was kicked out of her housing since she "smoked a cigarette on the balcony." After that, the court planned to place her in a local treatment center. There were no openings, so they sent her to jail for a month. Once completed, as Sarah told it, "drug court came in to see me. They made me sign this thing that said when I got out of jail—the only way I could get out of jail was to sign this paper that said I was not gonna get on any kind of opiates, no pain pills when I got out." She failed two subsequent outpatient drug tests and was terminated. She pled guilty and, as she had participated in drug court, received her full sentence of sixteen months.

William reasoned that being on drug court merely prolonged an inevitable sentence, so he sought to avoid the program altogether: "I would take jail before I would take drug court, honestly." Similarly, Nate felt that serving a sentence was easier than drug court participation:

> It's so much easier because I feel like they push you into doing a lot of things you don't want to do. It's a lot of pressure. If you don't do this, you get this. So why is that? . . . What if I don't want to do that? What if that's not my recovery?
>
> My recovery is different. My recovery is music. My recovery is writing and stuff like that—but not essays based on . . . what they put on you. And I knew that's what it entailed, so I was like, "Nah, I don't want to do that."

Kay, who had also been offered drug court, contended that the "program is made to set you up to fail." As she put it, "You can get more drugs in jail easier than in the streets, so why would you put an addict in jail while waiting to find a bed? You're setting them up to fail. . . . I just told them I'd rather sit in jail."

Mark had a more positive experience in the program. He felt supported by the team and developed trust with his therapist: "We have an understanding where she's not just gonna tell . . . drug court every little thing." He, however, recognized that, while drug court garnered him treatment resources, he needed criminal charges, or "legals," as interviewee Lisa had put it, to receive services: "I've only had the success I've had now because—a lot of it has to do with drug court, because there are certain doors that it opens up. You don't really sit on waiting lists very long when you're on drug court. . . . I am just doin' really well now, and the DA is part of that. They are on the drug court team. They are supportive of the program, and that's the aspect where that's nice. But on the other hand, I feel like I shouldn't have needed to get criminal charges to get help."

Conclusion: A Deadly Embrace

Whether an individual participant has a positive or negative experience, drug courts ultimately incorporate treatment within the criminal legal system. Treatment providers work with—or more accurately *for*—criminal courts. Therapeutic surveillance, which operates through a series of community nodes, is justified in drug court through participants adopting a liminal and racialized narrative identity: as "criminal addicts" (objects of control) destined for disposability and "recovering addicts" (objects of care) progressing toward freedom in productive citizenship, albeit often for low-wage labor.[56] Courtroom interaction, thus, *creates* the treatable carceral subject, while entrenching the criminal legal system within addiction recovery. While participants can resist drug court framings of addiction, or just go along with the program without personal investment, they are nevertheless confined to a drug court narrative habitus that is of material consequence.[57]

Taken together, drug courts perpetuate what Kerwin Kaye refers to as "caring violence," where "disciplinary measures are positioned as therapeutic and a form of help."[58] Caring violence is steeped in racist, patriarchal, and paternalistic control, as the benevolent patriarch asserts discipline to "lift[] the savage into a civilized state" through "a brutal hand" and "yielding heart."[59] Not just the appearance of benevolence, but empowerment discourses also compose caring violence. As Wendy Brown states, "empowerment is a formulation that converges with a regime's own legitimacy needs in masking the power of the regime."[60] After all, drug court sessions are not necessarily meant to be punishing but, as the city's website states, "a POSITIVE experience for team members and participants filled with smiles, applause and hope for each participants [*sic*] success."[61]

And, after graduation, participants remain suspect. Given "the idea that addiction is a chronic, relapsing disorder," as Rebecca Tiger reminds us, "'fixedness' is never assured and . . . long-term surveillance and coercion are therefore required."[62] Indeed, graduates often continue serving probation time, which puts them at risk of future incarceration. Such disciplinary practices also tie families into state surveillance.[63] Interviewee Michelle, a mother of the probationer Lucas, recounted an incident when a probation officer came in "screaming" during a random house visit. She reflected, "I'm not the one that's in trouble. Keep it down."[64] And, if the probationer violates, or "recidivates," they risk being incarcerated.[65] Rather than an alternative to jail, drug courts can be better understood as a fixture of a broader carceral circuit of care, in which criminal-justice-involved people find themselves—and their families—going in circles after arrest, moving between courts, treatment centers, jail, probation, restricted electronic monitoring, and back again.[66]

The overlap between drug court and jail proved deadly for forty-eight-year-old Rob Card. Card was arrested on January 8, 2017, and was incarcerated for a minor probation violation. The court placed him in jail while waiting for a treatment bed to open. He was being treated for a brain tumor and seizures, a fact known by police and court authorities. While incarcerated, he was denied medical care and was only given Tylenol. He was unable to walk, fell several times, and had ongoing seizures. He told his family over the phone, "Broome County is killing me." After thirteen days, Card was discharged and brought to the hospital in full seizure. He was kept on life support so he could donate his organs and died the next day.[67] His family met with the local organization Justice and Unity for the Southern Tier (JUST). Setting a container of his ashes on the meeting table, his sister declared, "Something really needs to be done about this."[68]

5

Caring Cages

Stories of Help and Harm

I am attending a rally at the Broome County Correctional Facility. It is during an open house event hosted by the sheriff. Participants are drawing attention to recent deaths in the facility, many the result of abuse by correctional officers and from poor medical care by the jail's private provider.

A few of the protesters, myself included, spray-painted a cardboard casket the previous night. It stands upright as cars drive by and attendees shout, "A jail sentence is not a death sentence!"

Several speak in front of the crowd. With megaphone in hand, an advocate tells of a young man who was incarcerated in the facility and had detoxed off of benzodiazepines and heroin. With no medical intervention, he had a seizure and was in a coma for ten days; he would require lifetime medication. A young woman steps to the median on an adjacent street. She tells of her experience detoxing in solitary confinement, while nervously—and bravely—sharing that it was only after she urinated herself that correctional officers let her out.[1]

While Southern Tier community members regularly documented harms at the jail, local officials continued to invest in the 536-bed facility.[2] As detailed in the introduction, in 2014 the county legislature passed a $6.8 million expansion, which converted a gymnasium into housing for incarcerated women, added a "new state-of-the-art medical unit," and reserved thirteen new deputy positions.[3] Between 2012 and 2023, the Broome County Sheriff's Office budget increased from $29.1 to $42.8 million, which took up roughly 10 percent of the budget. $31 million went to the facility, with the remaining going to county police.[4] In 2015, the jail had the second highest incarceration rate in New York State, only surpassed by Chemung County.[5]

Yet, such investment, as with police and court addiction treatment, was based not necessarily on "lock 'em up," tough-on-crime rhetoric but on addressing key issues that the protestors raised. The Republican sheriff, David Harder, assured that the new medical unit would be better equipped to handle incarcerated people with "heroin problems."[6] When announcing state funding for jail treatment in 2018, he claimed, as paraphrased by a reporter, "40 percent of inmates in the County Jail have a drug addiction problem. . . . This program is essential because it not only treats them while they are in jail, but also after they get out."[7] Republican State Senator Fred Akshar also appealed to a sympathetic view of incarcerated people who use drugs: "Anytime we can again get people into the road to recovery as quickly as possible, they become contributing members of society. It's incumbent upon us to provide the most basic of human services to people."[8] Meanwhile, the county cut mental and public health expenditures, with both offices taking up a combined 0.68 percent of the operating budget in 2023.[9] These budgetary decisions centralized county-funded health care within the jail.

While jail has been touted as a place of care, John Irwin contends that "the basic purpose of the jail is to manage society's rabble."[10] It is fitting, then, that the Broome County Correctional Facility sits on land formerly owned by the county's poor farm, the Broome County Almshouse, which held those who "were sick, disabled, mentally unwell, widowed, or orphaned, and they were expected to work on the farm and follow rigid rules for behavior."[11] In *The Jail Is Everywhere*, Jack Norton and fellow activists identify contemporary jails as holding federal and state prisoners as well as Immigration and Customs Enforcement (ICE) detainees, thus devolving federal and state authority to local actors.[12] Jails also contract with a variety of private providers—in commissary, food, medical care, and communication from phone calls, tablets, and electronic mail, all of which add to the sheriff's wallet.[13] To be sure, jails and prisons broaden racialized control, rooted in slavery, lynching, and Jim Crow segregation.[14] Despite this historical and structural context, jails and prisons have nevertheless been deemed as places of health-care and treatment support, particularly in response to the opioid crisis. In what ways does popular reporting on jail-based treatment justify carceral expansion? What are the experiences of incarcerated people who use drugs?

In this chapter, I explore popular *stories of carceral help* told by public officials, reporters, and some of those who had been incarcerated. These jail addiction-recovery narratives feature physically degraded "addicts" who, once incarcerated, seek recovery. Such stories, I argue, "repackage mass incarceration" by framing jails as "caring social service providers," as James Kilgore puts it when defining carceral humanism.[15] In contrast, I draw on *stories of carceral harm* told by formerly incarcerated interviewees who used opioids at the time of their arrest. Their experiences get to a deeper truth of jails—that they are fundamentally places of degradation and dehumanization through interpersonal and institutional violence. As the activist-scholar Hannah Walter reminds us, punitive health care cannot restore physical, mental, or emotional well-being and thus is not health care at all.[16]

Of significance, while those whom I interviewed were white, carceral harm is nevertheless an outgrowth of a carceral state rooted in anti-Black violence. As the "white addict" is a proxy for racialized insecurity, such punishment reinforces the ideals of white, middle-class citizenship, which the "white addict" has not achieved. And carceral punishment is against the backdrop of Black criminality. Indeed, in 2022, Black people made up 7 percent of the Broome County population but made up 35 percent of the jail population, and, in 2018, 97 percent of the correctional officers were white.[17] In turn, the disciplining of the Othered white subject, as "drug addict," reinforces the symbolic binary between white freedom and Black enslavement and monstrosity.[18] That is, state violence employed against Othered whites, as I have argued throughout this book, operates on the terrain of the color line, their symbolically possessed, trashed, criminalized, bestial, zombified, and enslaved bodies representing the racialized Other to be exorcised from white capitalist order, here in caring cages.

Stories of Carceral Help: "It Would Save His Life"

In *Dopesick*, Beth Macy offers the story of twenty-three-year-old Spencer Mumpower, who had used and dealt drugs in West Virginia. After selling the drug that resulted in his friend Scott Roth's overdose death, Mumpower was sentenced to eight years in prison. Macy describes his mug-shot photo: "His eyes are bruised and sunken, and there are chicken-pox-like scabs on his face—from the itch of amphetamines, of which he was also addicted. He weighed 135 pounds." His physical appearance was eye-opening. As he told Macy, "One day in jail I realized I could touch these two fingers around my forearm. . . . It meant I was a junkie." He desired change. As Macy adds, "After six months of begging for his mother to bail him out, he finally hit bottom and accepted he had nowhere to go but up." Mumpower committed to recovery, affirming to Macy, "I like being clean. I like being sober. I like being able to talk to my mother and she talks to me, and I get what's going on here." His counselor confirmed the positive role incarceration played in his recovery: "Fifteen rehabs had not convinced Spencer that it was not in his best interests to get high. It took time in jail and a friend dying before he could decide he wanted to change."[19] Macy concludes in earlier coverage that jail "would destroy Spencer's freedom, and ultimately, it would save his life."[20]

Numerous reporters offer such jail addiction-recovery narratives, of a criminal-justice-driven rock-bottom moment that is the catalyst for recovery.[21] Eric Eyre tells of Chelsea Carter, a "recovering 30-year-old addict" who worked as a therapist in a drug treatment center in Logan County, West Virginia. Carter quit taking opioids in 2008, on "the day she went to jail after taking part in a theft ring that sold stolen goods for painkillers." As she told Eyre, "When they handcuff you, and you walk through the doors, and you're in an orange jumpsuit and they slam the doors behind you, that's when you wonder, 'is two to 20 years worth it for one OxyContin?' . . . That's when I hit my knees and prayed, 'Lord, if you ever bring me out of this, I'll never touch another drug again.'"[22]

John Eaton offers the story of Austin Serb, a teenager who used and sold drugs. After a drug bust by the DEA, Serb was sentenced to ten years for conspiracy to distribute oxycodone. He sought change in prison, Eaton recounts. Serb "reads the bible everyday now. He is studying social psychology in college classes at the prison and tutors other prisoners who are studying for their GEDs." Eaton observes Serb's physical transformation: "It is a warm afternoon in April of 2017. Serb, now 24, wears khaki pants, a work shirt, and fashionable plastic-frame eyeglasses. His light brown hair is cropped close on the sides and slicked over in an aggressive part. Gone are the sunken, dark-rimmed eyes and pasty skin. He is up to 195 pounds, thanks to the days spent leading workouts in the prison gym. He is off drugs, which he says are widely available inside the prison, and his fidgety cooped-up energy is back." Eaton concludes, "Getting caught saved him. If Serb hadn't ended up in prison on federal drug charges, he says, he'd probably be dead too," referring to his friend who fatally overdosed.[23]

Jail addiction-recovery narratives tell not just of individual tenacity but of successful jail-based treatment initiatives. In Sam Quinones's book *The Least of Us* and in an opinion piece for *The New York Times*, he introduces Unit 104, a seventy-man pod established in 2015 in Kentucky's Kenton County jail. Quinones begins with a rock-bottom scenario: "In jail, detoxed of the dope that controlled their decisions on the street, addicts often behold the wreckage of their lives."[24] Subsequently, county jails "started full-time 'therapeutic communities' aimed at rehabilitation within their walls, providing inmates the services that private treatment centers offer on the outside."[25] In Unit 104, as Quinones continues participants provide peer support to challenge their "me-first criminal thinking." He adds, "Inmates governed themselves. One way they did this was by calling out each other for not putting forth their best effort, for getting up late, sleeping during the day, for lying or not making their bed. This went against everything that drug addiction and custody taught them. Dissolving the criminal code, learning to postpone immediate gratification and combat addiction—it all required using criticism to fuel personal change."[26] With such programming, Quinones adds, "Jail came to be seen as a necessary lever, a tool to force an addict to seek treatment before it was too late."[27]

Similarly, in *Raising Lazarus*, Beth Macy accounts for medication-assisted treatment (MAT) implementation in Virginia's Fairfax County Adult Detention Center. In the program, volunteers and public servants provide buprenorphine to incarcerated people, who are referred to as "individuals" or "members" instead of "inmates." This "lessen[s] stigma and create[s] buy-in and trust." For successful reentry, a peer support network coordinates housing and treatment services for a "'warm handoff' that facilitates continuing their bupe [buprenorphine]." This approach contrasts with the Surry County jail, where Macy witnessed incarcerated people puking in buckets in overcrowded cells. She thus deems Fairfax as "a law enforcement realm unto itself, a place where committed volunteers and public servants replaced Nancy Reagan's mantra with Shelly Young's," referring to a mother who began to view addiction as a medical condition after nearly losing her son.[28]

Jail addiction-recovery narratives consequently bolster sheriffs' and legislators' calls to increase jail funding on the basis of treatment support. The National Sheriffs' Association and the National Commission on Correctional Health Care asserted in 2018 that "[jails are in] a unique position to initiate treatment in a controlled, safe environment."[29] That same year, fifty-eight criminal justice officials, including current and former sheriffs, signed an open letter in support of MAT in jails, describing incarceration as a "pathway to treatment." The superintendent of the Cheshire County Department of Corrections in New Hampshire emphasized the social role jails play in the letter: "Society demands that [jails] also serve as a hospital, mental health institution, school and rehabilitation center."[30]

Ultimately, jail addiction-recovery narratives view jails as places of care. Rather than *extracting time*, as Ruth Wilson Gilmore argues of incarceration, jails ostensibly provide *life-sustaining recovery time*.[31] Certainly, incarcerated people deserve health-care access, including MAT, which has been shown to reduce fatal overdose rates upon release.[32] Furthermore, like drug court, incarceration *can be* motivation for some people to achieve desired abstinence and recovery. Interviewee Megan expressed that her sobriety was, in part, due to not wanting to be reincarcerated. She also felt more comfortable during her three months in jail than being in emergency housing or without shelter. As she put it, "It sounds crazy, but I was more comfortable where I was at in jail. I had my commissary. My parents were coming to see me. I was better off."[33]

Yet, given the structural conditions of incarceration within racial capitalism, it is misguided to view individual jail programs as benevolent law enforcement realms unto themselves. Even when referred to as "individuals" or "members" rather than "inmates," those who are incarcerated still arrive in handcuffs.[34] In the following section, I review experiences by formerly incarcerated interviewees who used drugs. Their stories encompass "a vast set of discarded experiences" across the jail's "abyssal divide," which separates those who are incarcerated from the community.[35] In offering their experiences, I hope not to reinforce the view of incarcerated people as passive objects of violence but to underscore "what's really going on" in the jail, to quote interviewee Ron.[36]

I also recognize interviewees' strength in sharing experiences of state violence. And, from their experiences, I find that jails are fundamentally places of dehumanization and degradation through interlocking interpersonal and institutional violence—comprising medical harm, gender and sexual harm, and reentry harm.

Medical Harm: "It's like an Insane Asylum"

Medical harm occurs through the jail's use of solitary confinement, punitive detox, and dangerous prescribing patterns and from harassment and physical abuse faced in the medical unit.

Nate accounted for isolation in the old medical unit, which had moldy mattresses and black mold in the showers. Correctional officers regularly denied phone access and recreational time, despite incarcerated people being guaranteed at least one hour of outdoor exercise daily.[37] "They tell you that you come out every twenty-three hours, you get an hour of rec, but they never send them out. Sometimes they would be in there for twenty-three days at a time and not even get an hour of rec. . . . It's like an insane asylum."

Lisa spent six days in solitary confinement, where she detoxed off heroin. She spoke of being harassed by a correctional officer: "With me, I was going through the worst detox of my life, and they gave me Motrin [a minor painkiller]. Sometimes they'll check on you, and I'll be passed out on the floor, like completely passed out. They'll bang on the door [and ask], 'You alive?' 'Yes.' And they would kind of harass me, be like, 'How are those fuckin' drugs treating you now?'"

Hannah documented her experience of "absolute withdrawal" in a neighboring jail, where she spent seven business days in medical confinement: "Not only was I coming off of Suboxone cold turkey; I was coming off of all my depression meds, anxiety meds, hormones. . . . I was a fuckin' wreck. . . . I wrote a suicide letter to my kids. I had a plan picked out. I knew I was doing it and that I was ending it. I couldn't take it anymore."

Sarah spoke of isolation and a lack of medication access. She was incarcerated for a drug court violation and was placed in solitary confinement. She broke four of her vertebrae from a fall three weeks prior and was wearing a back brace. She spent twenty-one days in isolation.

They left me in there. I didn't even get "rec." I was locked in twenty-four hours a day. . . . And they only would let me have one mattress, and I was supposed to have two. The mattresses are this thin [indicates a small height with her hands]. I'm sleeping on concrete with a broken back. It was so bad, I had to sleep with my back brace on.

. . . That's when I was, like, paralyzed, and I peed myself and they left me. So, finally, after the twenty-one days or whatever, I got cleared by medical to be released.

In the general population, Sarah had reoccurring foot issues: "My foot kept swelling really huge, and it was purple, and I couldn't walk." She was escorted to the medical unit but did not receive her prescriptions.

So they walked me down to medical one day because of my foot, and they refused to see me. They were like, "No. We're not seeing you. We're not gonna do anything for you." They sent me back. I was crying all night, because it hurt—my back hurt, everything.

. . . They wouldn't let me have my prescriptions. That's one thing that's really fucked up, because I came in with current prescriptions.

Ron, who was unhoused at the time of our interview, offered a myriad of abuses, including solitary confinement, poor detox, use of restraint chairs, harassment, physical abuse, and family disconnection:

I was withdrawing from heroin [due to "a bad batch that was going around at the time"], and I was stuck in a medical observation cell. . . . I kept having what [the correctional officers] were calling "pseudo-seizures." That's all that was explained to me. They induced me in a coma, and I was brought back and forth from the hospital to the jail . . . multiple times. My family tried calling the jail to see if I was still in their custody. The jail said that I was no longer in their custody.

. . . I kept having seizures in there. They thought I was faking 'em, so they kept stomping, they stomped on my hand. . . . They thought by stomping on my hand it would get me to wake up from my seizure and admit, "Oh, I'm faking it." So they did that. They really hurt my hand pretty bad.

. . . I had another seizure, and they swore that I was faking it, so they— they stripped me butt naked [and] strapped me to a restraint chair for a couple days [in the medical unit]. The corrections officer [who knew Ron's family] said, "You know your own parents want nothing to do with you. You can't work for your father's company because you're such a heroin addict, you piece of shit. . . . We know you're faking your seizures. You're a fucking scumbag. . . . All you're doing is causing taxpayers more money. . . . You know, we ought to just let you die in a cell. It would cost everybody less money."

. . . Even when I wasn't having seizures and stuff, they kept breaking them ["old-school ammonia sticks"] underneath my nose, and [they were] basically torturing me with them just because I couldn't move, you know, I could barely move my head. . . . They weren't really letting me eat much of anything. They're giving me juice cups, that's it. They weren't letting me eat meals. They weren't letting me use the bathroom or anything like that.

. . . They [eventually] sent me to the box. . . . I was tortured in the box basically more or less every day. A CO came in by the name of "Grasshopper" and would literally beat the living shit out of me.

. . . They withheld my visits. They withheld my phone calls. . . . [My] family wouldn't even know what was going on because anytime they came for a visit, they would say, "Oh, no, he's not in the box anymore because there's special visiting hours for the box." . . . I was trying to send out letters to my family to say, "Get a hold of an attorney," stuff like that so people can know what's going on. I assume my letters never reached home or anything like that.

Harm takes on explicit racist dimensions for incarcerated people of color. Lawsuits reveal the particularly racist abuse that two Black men faced by correctional officers. In 2015, thirty-six-year-old Salladin Barton died after the jail doctor prescribed two counteracting drugs.[38] He was also starved and beaten by officers who directed racial epithets at him, as an incarcerated witness recounted:

Correctional officer(s) . . . beat Mr. Barton continuously and even bust his head open so he had to get staples in his head. . . . And the day before he died they ran in his cell and beat him up again. I could hear the CO yelling "I'm a kill you N****r, I'm a kill you n***a." When they left his cell I ask him is he ok and he told me he was dizzy and bleeding in his head. . . .

The very next day . . . he said he feels dizzy. I told him to lay down and that's when . . . I heard the thump. . . . I begin to call his name loudly and he would not respond.[39]

Black and Latinx nineteen-year-old Taej'on Vega also documented in a legal complaint that he was denied four prescribed drugs. During a "shakedown," officers beat, strip-searched, and harassed him, threatening, "You're not so tough are you," "I don't [want to] hear a peep out of you now," and "Do what you're told n****r."[40]

Interviewees and legal cases speak to two dimensions of carceral harm. First, there are *interpersonal* violations of protected standards of care: of denying recreation and phone time and of harassment and physical abuse. There are also forms of *institutionalized* violence that nevertheless fulfill standards of care. In the new medical unit, incarcerated people sit in isolated cells, where lights are left on and the temperature is not controlled, which "assault[s] the senses with oppressive effects."[41] Incarcerated people can be made to wait up to fourteen days for medication, and the jail's physician can over- and underprescribe original doses.[42] Indeed, the formal intake process is itself punishing. A formerly incarcerated trans activist interviewee, Imani, spoke of the intake process in the men's unit: It involves the taking of property, fingerprinting and mug shots, and movement in and out of the crowded "clinical bullpen," the latter echoing the confinement of a slave pen.[43] Constant moving *and* waiting causes disorientation and is itself dehumanizing.[44] Such practices in turn constitute what John Irwin refers to as "mortifying rituals," which include "the searching, stripping, bathing, spraying, and the taking of personal property [which] are conducted with the institutional purpose of converting newcomers into manageable inmates."[45] Interpersonal and institutional harms are further evident in gender and sexual violence.

Gender and Sexual Harm: "It Was the Worst Experience of My Life"

Interviewees, advocates, and lawsuits reveal the scope of gender and sexual violence in jail, including voyeurism, strip searches, and sexual harassment and assault.

In the local *Press & Sun-Bulletin*, advocates Judy Arnold and Alexis Pleus wrote of a lack of privacy in the new women's dormitory:

> It is a giant former gymnasium where everything is in the same room. . . . Women sleep in bunks along the walls, eat in the middle of the room at tables just several feet from their beds, shower in stalls with no shower curtain and use open toilets with no walls around them, next to each other and within eyeshot of where people sit to eat. . . . Along another wall are showers with a door so small that it may cover both your breasts and privates if you're the optimal height, but one inch taller or shorter, and you are fully exposed.
>
> . . . Imagine trying to use the bathroom while all your bunkmates and corrections officers can see you. Imagine being a woman menstruating and having to tend to your female needs while people can watch you.[46]

Lisa confirmed this lack of privacy in our interview: "In the new pod, the bathrooms are like here. The CO's desk was here [hand motions indicate a close proximity]. Yeah, it's uncomfortable. . . . Even in the other pod that I'm usually in [the old dorm pod], the showers' stalls are here, and the COs' desks are here, and the shower stalls were like that long [indicates a small length]." Indeed, such voyeurism is a matter of policy, with the jail handbook stating, "Officers of both genders supervise inmates in housing areas. It *is your responsibility* to maintain your privacy within limits of security. No inmate is allowed to obstruct the view of the cell, shower, windows or other area with any item."[47]

Such voyeurism is indicative of an environment conducive to sexual violence and harassment.[48] Lisa offered an instance of harassment by a correctional officer: "There's this one CO, he would come into our pod and scream, 'Free heroin!' Or when we would go to the library, he'd be like, 'Oh, you guys going to get free drugs?' . . . He would go into the pod—there's a lot of prostitution going on, you know, with drugs and stuff like that. He would start laying out hundreds on the table and then be like, 'Ladies, I haven't even gotten paid yet' . . . And, like, a lot of 'em turned tricks, and a lot of 'em take advantage of that." At times, advances are less explicit, as Lisa explained:

There were a couple of girls that would stay up at night, and the COs would come around and kind of flirt with 'em, hit on 'em, and stuff like that. It was just, it was gross. . . . They pass notes and stuff like that. . . . One of the COs, we used to get into hockey a lot, and he slid a note underneath my mattress, and I was like, "What the fuck?" I thought maybe it was from somebody else, like in a different pod. It was from him. . . . It said something about, "We should watch the game sometime." And I'm like, "If I write back to this, this is going to end up being something." . . . "I can make your stay better or worse"—I've seen a lot of that.

Sexual violence is not restricted to interpersonal harassment but also includes standardized strip searches. As Angela Davis argues, "The state itself is directly implicated in this routinization of sexual abuse, both in permitting such conditions that render women vulnerable to explicit sexual coercion carried out by guards and other prison staff and by incorporating into routine policy such practices as the strip search and body cavity search."[49] Keri Blakinger reports in her memoir, *Corrections in Ink*, on a strip search her unit faced during a retaliatory shakedown in a New York prison. During one incident, "there was a new twist: If you were on your period, you had to take out your bloody tampon and put it on the floor so the guard could be sure you were not smuggling anything back from your visit."[50] Makyyla Holland, a Black transgender woman, documented her experience at the Broome County jail for the New York Civil Liberties Union: "I was humiliated by Broome County jail staff because I am a transgender woman. I was harassed, mocked, misgendered and worse: jail staff strip-searched me, beat me up, placed me in the male section of the jail, and withheld my hormones for a period of time, forcing me to go into agonizing withdrawal."[51] Such abuse, to be sure, compounds past trauma that so many incarcerated women and gender-nonconforming people have experienced.

Incarcerated pregnant women face particular scrutiny, given Western ideals of motherhood and "true womanhood."[52] Interviewee Elizabeth documented her experiences in the jail. We talked in her living room as her daughter played with a spatula. "I was pregnant. I was pregnant with her. When I went there, I was coming off drugs, and I was sick, and they could put you on methadone [for pregnant people], and that's how I got on methadone. But initially, before they did that, they were, like, just telling me how—a nurse there told me how I deserved to go to hell because I was pregnant and using drugs and how I'm a terrible person, how I didn't deserve to have children." A correctional officer added, "You don't deserve to have a child. I honestly hope that child dies in your stomach because you're gonna have another addict baby who is just like you." Elizabeth concluded, "It was the worst experience of my life."

Incarceration furthermore separates parent and child. It produces what Mariame Kaba calls "un-mothering," which refers to "the ways the state and society actively and violently threaten, remove, disappear, and kill Black women's children."[53] Un-mothering is rooted in chattel slavery and colonial conquest and is built into contemporary forms of incarceration, drug war, and government child removal.[54] Un-mothering is constitutive of "natal alienation," as Joshua Price puts it in his collaborative jail research: "Jails and prisons offer substandard and indifferent prenatal care, shackle pregnant women, and separate mothers and their children. . . . The state dictates whether and how one is allowed to parent. . . . Tracing the history of natal alienation shows how the forced separation of incarceration echoes that of slavery."[55] Certainly, carceral violence can lead to miscarriage; this is un-mothering prior to a child's birth, or perhaps a more accurate term might be involuntary *non*-mothering.[56]

To reiterate, violence against women and gender-nonconforming people flows out of the long-standing treatment of incarcerated women of color; it is built on a legacy of colonialism, slavery, and segregation.[57] The harms of incarceration are therefore exacerbated for people who use drugs and have faced socially structured inequality, including for Black, Indigenous, and Chicanx women and gender-nonconforming people.[58] And, to be sure, all violence within white supremacist capitalist patriarchy is raced and gendered, including the misogynistic emasculation inherent in male strip searches in prisons and jails and in police stop-and-frisks that involve "the spreading of the legs and the groping of the thighs and genitals."[59] Harms continue upon release, including increased risks of fatal overdose.

Reentry Harm: "The Clean Time Is What Kills People"

Those who are released from incarceration have a heightened risk of overdose. Researchers have attributed this to reduced tolerance upon release and to a punitive and nonresponsive reentry system.[60]

Reduced tolerance can be particularly risky for those who use intravenously. Jim put it this way in our interview: "The clean time is what kills people, bro. . . . You get a big-ass gap, and you go right back to the needle. I only met one person my entire life who shot up instantly. . . . You gotta graduate into the needle."[61] Vincent determined that lowered tolerance from jail incarceration contributed to his cousin's postrelease fatal overdose: "He [the drug dealer his cousin was working for] was a real big player. . . . My cousin was evidently selling for him. They [police] picked him up on somethin' minor, locked his ass in jail, and just tried to talk him into snitching. He wouldn't do it, so he spends a week in jail, and he's pretty much going through hell, but still, not even remotely off the drugs [in the sense of quitting]. I think he did a six- or eight-bag hit, first thing . . . when he got home, and he died."

Reentry death is also a consequence of a punitive and nonresponsive reentry system. Incarceration disrupts employment and social service access.[62] In Broome County, it can take up to thirty to forty-five days to receive benefits from the Department of Social Services (DSS) and up to five days to access the expedited Supplemental Nutrition Assistance Program (SNAP), or "food stamps."[63] In 2022, it took an average of fifty-nine days for a Broome County resident to receive SNAP benefits.[64] Since many counties do not allow incarcerated people to apply for DSS from prison or jail, this leaves a dangerous gap.[65] Interviewee Sarah reapplied for Medicaid after nine months of being incarcerated. She was released on August 10 but had to wait until September 1 to receive health insurance. The jail let her leave with her psychiatric medication but withheld medication she used to manage epileptic seizures. "And you detox from that," she added, "It was horrible."

To receive services, one must also manage DSS appointments. As Mary, a peer reentry coordinator, stated for those who are recently released, "They have to go to DSS the very next morning. If they don't have a ride, they've gotta take all their crap with them, all their belongings. . . . A lot of times people don't make the meetings, so then they have to start—their forty-five-day wait starts all over again [Mary is referring to the application period to receive safety net assistance (SNA)]. So then they end up in situations where they don't have any place to go."[66] As we spoke at a diner, Mary revealed the dizzying lengths one must go to in order to access services, food, emergency housing, clothing, personal care items, and communication devices:

> You're sitting in each place. It's not like you have a 10:30 appointment, and you get in at 10:30 and be out of there at 10:15 or 10:45. That's not happening. When I take people to go apply for the emergency housing and their SNAP, their food stamps, I usually pick them up from jail after 10:00. I tell them, "I'm here to pick up so-and-so." They'll say, "Wait in your car. They'll be discharged." And they're discharged.
>
> Sometimes they have a bag of clothing; sometimes they have nothing. And so we go directly to the Department of Social Services, and if they're literate and don't need the help, I have them fill out the application on the way down. If not, we go down there, we turn it in, and then they say, "You gotta come back at 1:00," 'cause that's when they'll process. They'll try to find emergency housing for them and all that.
>
> So after I leave there, then we go to the clothing bank, if they need clothes. We go to Ladies of Charity Clothing, and then I go to the homeless outreach worker, 'cause when they apply for SNAP, even though they have no money—the expedited SNAP—people call it "emergency SNAP," but it's "expedited." They have one to five days to issue that allotment. It never happens in one. It's two to five.
>
> So I go to the homeless outreach worker, and she usually gives me gift cards for people to eat—Subway, New York Pizza, McDonald's—so they have something to eat waiting for their SNAP to come in. We can go to food pantries or community meals if they're close to some. They have some every day of the week, but they're all over the county. . . .
>
> But we can go to the food pantry. If they're somewhere like the single-room housing, they have a shared kitchen, but you might not have any pots and pans to cook. So usually when we go to the food pantry for emergency food, we'll get peanut butter and jelly or ramen noodles, if they have it, whatever—something they could do relatively—without pots and pans and all that other stuff and refrigeration.

Then, after I take them to get the food coupons from the homeless outreach worker and the clothing bank, then we go to United Presbyterian Church to get personal care items. We have it worked out. They have a program called Care and Share that gives you items that you cannot buy with SNAP—so toothbrushes, razors, shaving cream, body soap, dish soap, laundry detergent, toilet paper, stuff like that.

And then I have a little bit of money that I have to try to decide, "What is most important for you? What do you really need?" So a lot of times, it's spent, like—they'll go into the single-room housing, and I'll end up buying—they have a blowup mattress that usually goes flat. I usually end up buying them sheets and a pillow and blankets. I have some stored up, so I'm good on that, and I try to get them a telephone 'cause they have to communicate with me. And they may have probation, drug and alcohol treatment, set up appointments, so I try to get them a telephone.

Now the thing with the free phones through Assurance Wireless, you have to have an address and a photo ID, and you have to have a SIM number, so you have to have a benefit card with a SIM number on it, 'cause they bill it, and most people don't have that. So sometimes I'll have to go, and I'll have to buy them a phone and a phone card, and that ends up to be $75. That's a lot of money out of—all's I got allotted for them is $104.

And then when thirty days are up, or who knows how long that the phone card's gonna last. It's 350 minutes and one thousand texts or something, but they blow through that, and so it's tough. It's tough trying to get all their needs met with the little bit of money that I have for each person.

From this, one can see how the welfare system—whether accessed by those who are formerly incarcerated or not—*is policing*, as it disciplines, regulates, and punishes.[67]

As evident in Mary's account, not only are services hard to access, but they are often inadequate. Carl was incarcerated for a non-drug-related offense, which cost him his construction job. Upon release, he was placed in emergency housing. He described it as a "shithole": "It's a rooming house, drug infested, guns, three ODs [overdoses] in one week, cops there every night." Advocate Erika offered an instance when someone she was supporting was not able to access a domestic, or intimate partner, violence shelter unless they detoxed off methamphetamine, but there was no such detox in the area. Another client of hers was put in emergency housing "right down the street from where she used to buy all her drugs." In addition, state-certified residential centers, which are apartments with added services like "managed healthcare and monthly welfare stipends," have also expelled people in recovery by labeling them as "treatment clients" and not "residents" who have tenant rights.[68]

Reentry services also do not speak to the on-the-ground needs of incarcerated people. Programming tends to focus on skill development and behavioral modification related to parenting, anger management, and employability.[69] Programs emphasize "grit," "moral redemption," "enhanc[ing] personal qualities," and "introspective work," rather than addressing structural circumstances and personal needs.[70] As Reuben Miller contends in *Halfway Home*, "As long as formally incarcerated people are legally excluded from the labor and housing markets, investing in their human capital won't do much to improve their lives. Reentry organizations can't erase their records or change their social situations."[71] When one does receive work, it is often in a precarious, low-wage labor market, where they are subjected to workplace humiliation and hyper-exploitation, as Gretchen Purser found when interviewing clients in a Syracuse, New York, reentry program.[72] Furthermore, reentry's focus on recidivism and enhancing public safety prioritizes, as Joshua Price puts it, "reoffending over advocacy."[73] A focus on recidivism, then, operates for the *threat management* of offenders. In this regard, those who are reentering bear what Rueben Miller and Forrest Stuart refer to as "carceral citizenship," as "a distinct form of political membership."[74]

To be sure, public officials regularly expressed concern about postincarceration overdoses, particularly when supporting jail and reentry treatment access. In advocating for jail treatment and reentry outpatient care, the Republican Broome County district attorney, Steve Cornwell, stated in a Broome Opioid Awareness Council (BOAC) meeting that when it comes to people overdosing upon release, "for those who don't think it is real, it is."[75] The county's emergency medical services (EMS) coordinator further stated in our interview, "I think the highest goal for the criminal justice system should be guiding people effectively toward treatment and recovery. . . . It pains me to know that people are sitting in jail going through painful withdrawal, and they're not really doing anything for them. Is that really necessary, you know?" When supporting treatment access inside and outside the jail, the DSS/mental health commissioner added in our interview, "Because we know that when addicts go to jail, if they don't get treatment, if they don't start on something, they go out, and they have such a high rate of dying the next time they use, because their bodies aren't used to—because they haven't used, and then they go use again, and they think they can use as much as they— and then they die."

Nevertheless, postincarceration treatment access does not necessarily result in fewer arrests or less incarceration, nor does it fundamentally alter the largely punitive reentry system. Rather, reentry treatment fashions the jail as the primary point of contact for services. Even as officials criticized the conditions of incarceration and reentry in the community, they promoted efforts that would further centralize services within the criminal legal system. And ongoing investment in the criminal legal system ultimately contributes to risks of overdose.[76] Perhaps it is more accurate to say here that it is not so much the "clean time" that kills people but *doing time* that does so.

Conclusion: "No More Jail Deaths"

Stories of carceral help and stories of carceral harm contrast strikingly. Consider Quinones's reporting of Unit 104 against interviewees' experiences:

> QUINONES: "Jail can be a necessary, maybe the only, lever with which to encourage or force an addict who has been locked up to seek treatment before it's too late."
>
> INTERVIEWEES: "We ought to just let you die in a cell" (Ron); "I wrote a suicide letter to my kids" (Hannah); "There's a lot of prostitution going on" (Lisa).
>
> QUINONES: "Once in custody and detoxed of the dope that has controlled their decisions, it's in jail where addicts more clearly behold the wreckage of their lives."
>
> INTERVIEWEES: "They would kind of harass me, be like, 'How are those fuckin' drugs treating you now?'" (Lisa); "They told me my baby's going to be an addict" (Elizabeth).

QUINONES: "County jails . . . have started full-time 'therapeutic communities' aimed at rehabilitation within their walls, providing inmates the services that private treatment centers offer on the outside."
INTERVIEWEES: "I'm sleeping on concrete with a broken back" (Sarah); "[The medical unit] is like an insane asylum" (Nate); "[T]hey stripped me butt naked [and] strapped me to a restraint chair for a couple days" (Ron).[77]

While incarceration does help some people seek a desired state of recovery, interviewees' experiences speak to jails as places of dehumanization and degradation, generated through interpersonal and institutional violence.[78] Even when "inmates" are referred to as "individuals" in need of help, incarcerated people are still deemed untrustworthy and are ridiculed, demeaned, and regulated.[79] Instead of places of health care, prisons and jails make people sicker and exacerbate preexisting health conditions, increasing risks of heart disease, cancer, and suicide.[80] As Rose Braz of Critical Resistance has put it, "Prisons and horrible conditions go hand in hand. The prison industrial complex (PIC) systematically undermines the very values and things we need to be healthy."[81]

As a final note, it is important to consider how appeals to legal rights to provide MAT in jails, such as the Americans with Disabilities Act (ADA), still permit the criminalization of people who use drugs and disabled people more generally.[82] While police are not constitutionally permitted to arrest someone for being "addicted to the use of narcotics," they can—and certainly do—for drug possession.[83] This effectively means that police can legally arrest people for expressing symptoms of SUD. After all, a symptom of opioid use disorder (OUD) is *obtaining* (i.e., *possessing*) opioids.[84] The language of rights therefore sets the groundwork to *take away* rights through arrest, incarceration, and accommodation. After all, police do not arrest people with diabetes for insulin possession, with the benevolent promise of that same insulin waiting for them behind bars.[85] People with SUD, who are at risk of being arrested for drug possession, also disproportionately have co-occurring disorders including anxiety and mood disorders, schizophrenia, bipolar disorder, major depressive disorder, conduct disorders, posttraumatic stress disorder, and attention deficit hyperactivity disorder.[86] Ongoing policing of possession, even with MAT protections, means that disabled people will continue to be, as Talila Lewis puts it, "primary among the carceral machine's intended targets."[87]

Even when accommodations are mandated, it does not mean that people who are incarcerated will receive them or that they will be allocated in a nonpunitive manner. Spencer Norris interviewed formerly incarcerated people who participated in the state-mandated MAT program in the Broome County jail. Interviewee Joshua Cotrill did not receive medication until he suffered from severe withdrawal symptoms: "[He] became so sick that when he tried to walk, he passed out, falling and hitting his head on the floor. Staff removed him in a wheelchair. He started the MOUD [medications for opioid use disorder] program the next day." Once in the program, participants were required to line up daily at 4:30 a.m. to receive eight- to sixteen-milligram doses, which may not have been enough for those with higher tolerances. Jail staff also switched interviewee Keith Keefe from prescribed methadone to buprenorphine. Keefe stated in dismay, "I'm like a potential walking overdose waiting to happen."[88] In addition, those who smuggle buprenorphine into the jail are at risk of being criminally charged.[89] To be sure, the jail's use of buprenorphine also drives pharmaceutical profitability, with buprenorphine being a ready-made market solution for a captive consumer base.[90]

It is imperative that people who are incarcerated receive health-care support and accommodation. Yet, as Ruth Wilson Gilmore and Craig Gilmore remind us, "legal protections under the law are not protections *from* the law."[91] After all, police prioritize order, not law, and rights have long facilitated state domination.[92] The polio survivor, author, and activist Judy Heumann puts it this way: "It's one thing to have our rights, but that doesn't mean you have justice."[93] To advocate for health-care support inside and outside the criminal legal system without reproducing that very same system, we need what the abolitionists Mariame Kaba and Kelly Hayes refer to as a "jailbreak of the imagination."[94]

In returning to the jail protest that I opened this chapter with, I view the action as ongoing communal resistance against localized drug war and mass incarceration. The casket, the speakers, and the banners are in place, as protestors participate in the theaters of meaning in which resistance plays out.[95] A photograph sits on my bookshelf as I write this, gifted by a fellow activist. In it, I am holding a banner with the text, "No

More Jail Deaths." Two people stand by my side. One has since passed away, and we continue to carry his spirit with us. And he continues to prop us up. I feel empowered in resistance—in local action against the jail, as an institution predicated on human debasement, humiliation, and interpersonal and institutional violence. In the conclusion, I reflect on such actions as local efforts to oppose carceral care—based on the caring violence of cops, courts, and cages—for a new ethic of care: abolitionist care.

Conclusion

Toward Abolitionist Care

I opened this book with an excerpt from Laura's drug court graduation. Onstage, she announced that from court-based treatment she regained custody of her child. She declared, "This is proof that God works in mysterious ways. The arrest saved my life. Angels come in black and blue clothes."[1] Interviewee Megan felt that, while certainly a difficult experience, incarceration was "more comfortable" than being in emergency housing or being unhoused. Her desire not to be reincarcerated also motivated her recovery, which was aided by drug court participation. Another criminal justice success story is that of Misti Barrickman, who was documented by Maia Szalavitz in *Unbroken Brain*. Barrickman was "homeless and addicted to heroin" before entering Law Enforcement Addiction Diversion (LEAD). Once incarcerated, she pleaded with the sergeant "to give her a chance to get treatment." Against policy, he permitted her access and directed her to a methadone appointment. Szalavitz updates the reader, "Set free and helped to start medication, she is now in college and has more than two years in recovery."[2] These stories, as evident in my fieldwork and in reporting, are a testament to the role that criminal justice actors can play in people's lives.

Yet, while some people may receive support, carceral care, by police, courts, and jailers, largely upholds a punitive criminal legal system rooted in racial capitalism—which is ultimately harmful for all. Through policing treatment, police gatekeep health-care access and deputize social workers to monitor participants. Police diversion programs can also rely on drug forfeiture funds and on people seeking treatment as confidential informants. Drug treatment courts enact therapeutic surveillance, which overlaps treatment providers and criminal justice actors in drug testing, coerced counseling, and electronic monitoring. Drug court participants, too, are made to adopt a bifurcated addiction identity, as "criminal addicts" and "recovering addicts," who are deemed to require the caring and controlling violence of the state. Jail treatment furthermore centralizes health care within the criminal legal system, as one must be incarcerated to access services at all. Those who are incarcerated then face interpersonal and institutional violence, from strip searches, harassment, physical abuse, and solitary confinement. Criminal-justice-based treatment, while appearing benevolent and perhaps an "ethically acceptable" form of punishment, ultimately bolsters mass incarceration, mass supervision, and mass policing, here in the Southern Tier of New York, a region marked by deindustrialization, poverty, and job loss.[3]

Carceral treatment is made sensible, as I have argued, through a dominant social problem representation of addiction as a disease, in particular through the popularized depiction of the white opioid user. While potentially humanizing, language and imagery of addicted bodies and brains, as apparent in brain scans, diagnostic criteria, and despair discourse, tell of drug-addicted whites transforming into metaphorical zombies, beasts, and slaves, which are indicative of racialized Otherness. Treatment subsequently operates through disciplinary regimes to restore order, largely through criminal justice intervention. Contra the "opioid user," the stereotypical "opioid dealer" is a violent, profiteering Black outsider who wreaks havoc in, and is meant to be expelled from, the (white) community. A popularized user/dealer divide thus permits policing through public health and suppression through drug raids and gang takedowns. Since security is never fully achievable, the fear of racialized disorder, evoked through the social problem formula stories of the medicalized addict and the menacing dealer, ensures ongoing drug war—and ever-mounting overdose deaths.

Despite that prohibition does not reduce the supply of or demand for drugs and even increases the risks of drug use, reporters and advocates have maintained faith in benevolent cops, courts, and cages. While one treatment-based reform may not work, there always appears another carceral fix. While Szalavitz compellingly argues in *Unbroken Brain* against drug criminalization and drug courts, she praises LEAD as "not punitive."[4] In downtown Seattle, Szalavitz contends, "LEAD officers are no longer the enemy."[5] In *Raising Lazarus*, Beth Macy critiques drug court for being expensive and run by nonspecialist court actors. Still, she trumpets jail-based treatment and promotes collaboration between advocates and criminal justice actors for progressive drug policy.[6]

Certainly, people need access to health care, inside and outside the criminal legal system. So, we may ask, "Isn't something better than nothing?" Yet, as Maya Schenwar and Victoria Law remind us, "In so many cases, reform is not the building of something new. It is the re-forming of the system in its own image, using the same raw materials: white supremacy, a history of oppression, and a tool kit whose main contents are confinement, isolation, surveillance, and punishment."[7] Carceral concessions that deem one criminal justice program as better than another simply do not amount to justice—and, in fact, double down on the systemic conditions that produce harm in the first place.[8] As Mariame Kaba puts it, "a gentler prison and policing system cannot adequately address harms," and as Alex Vitale adds, "a kinder, gentler, and more diverse war on the poor is still a war on the poor."[9]

Instead of reformist carceral concessions that entrench police power in the lives and bodies of people who use and deal drugs—and all of us, whether one uses or deals drugs or not—we need to abolish carceral care and replace it with abolitionist care.

Imagining and Doing Abolitionist Care

In *Let This Radicalize You*, Kelly Hayes and Mariame Kaba define abolition as "a broad-ranging movement to eradicate the prison-industrial complex and its foundations of racial capitalism, settler colonialism, and cis-hetero-patriarchy."[10] Abolitionists focus not on reforming the criminal legal system but on dismantling it altogether. As per this definition, abolitionists recognize that the criminal legal system is embedded within racial capitalism, so tweaks, or even governmental overhauls, do not fundamentally alter capitalism's basic drive for "accumulation for the sake of accumulation."[11] It is, after all, a system organized through a police-backed market bent, not on social need but profitability. In whatever form it takes, including the yearned-for welfare capitalism of Broome County past, capitalism necessarily produces exploitation, alienation, poverty, climate collapse, and crises.

Abolitionists do not reject reform entirely. Rather, they promote nonreform reforms, or abolitionist reforms, that "reduce rather than strengthen the scale and scope of policing, imprisonment, and surveillance."[12] As Rachel Herzing has it, abolition requires "being mindful not to build something today that will need to be torn down later on the path toward the long-term goal."[13] This means rejecting reforms that add funding to and a reliance on police through technology and community-oriented approaches.[14] Abolitionists do support campaigns at the international, national, state, and local levels, such as to end solitary confinement, life in prison without parole (LWOP), mandatory minimums, and death penalty sentencing. They also mobilize to defund police; close down, decarcerate, and prevent the expansion of jails, prisons, and all manner of carcerality, including e-monitoring devices and coerced treatment; and break the links between prisons/jails and ICE, US marshals, and private companies.[15]

In these efforts, abolitionists recognize the humanity of incarcerated people who do not fit the "relatively innocent" nonviolent, nonserious, nonsexual offender category.[16] Indeed, in critiquing the drug war, reporters and advocates have upheld the role of police for "serious crimes." Ryan Hampton argues in *Fentanyl Nation* that if we defelonize drug use and simple possession, police can "focus on more serious crimes" like "property crimes and violence."[17] Similarly, in *War on Us*, Colleen Cowles argues that ending the drug war will allow "police [to] be able to more effectively focus on solving violent crime like rape, murder, armed robbery, and assault."[18] While these writers speak to certainly harmful actions, such assertions of police presume that they do indeed make communities safe and that incarceration reduces harm and violence. Such a commitment to policing also fuels retributive justice, which produces, as Achille Mbembe contends, "endless reprisals, vengeance, and revenge."[19] To be sure, even prosecuting physicians and pharmaceutical actors does not fundamentally alter the institutions or industries that these actors are born out of.[20]

But there is a second part to the definition that is just as important as the first: Abolition involves "creat[ing] new systems in its [the prison industrial complex's] place that focus on meeting people's needs, preventing and transforming harm, and building true community safety and well-being."[21] In short, *tearing down requires building up.*[22] This necessitates thinking outside of jails and prisons as catch-all solutions to social problems.[23] Abolitionists have supported government funding for public education, affordable housing, labor protections, universal basic income, free child-care access, reproductive rights, reparations, and universal health care.[24] Building up cannot rely on pressing government spending alone. Rather, abolitionists recognize the importance of mutual aid, as "collective and community-based practices and efforts to meet people's needs, independent of state systems and other hierarchical, oppressive arrangements."[25] Mutual aid was readily practiced, for example, when protestors shared masks, food, medical support, physical protection, and shelter during the 2020 George Floyd uprisings. Abolition also encompasses direct action, restorative and transformative justice, and the creation of defense committees and conflict, deescalation, and community safety strategies.[26] Thus, while the term "crisis" connotes a need for police, especially when applied to a particular drug, people *do* show up with generosity and care in times of crises—and crises, too, reveal a rupture in current social and economic relations that can be a catalyst for action.[27] As Stuart Hall has stated of crisis, "It's the moment when you can raise deeper institutional questions, the moment when you can actually change something."[28]

In adopting an abolitionist approach, Black activists, scholars, and writers have supported healing justice. Erica Woodland describes healing justice as building an ecology of care by drawing on spiritual technologies that "our ancestors" adopted "as part of their overall strategies for liberation."[29] Alexis Pauline Gumbs conjures the spirit of Harriet Tubman navigating fire, sky, water, and earth to guide herself and others to freedom.[30] When traveling out of the Southern slave states, Tubman gave opioids to infants and children so they could sleep and be carried on the journey—that is abolitionist health care.[31] Formerly enslaved Africans developed Maroon communities, which included some Indigenous people and even white indentured servants.[32] Restorative justice, which views harm as a violation of interpersonal relationships and involves community engagement as a response, has roots in Indigenous practices.[33] The Black Panthers, too, implemented "free breakfast programs, bus rides, ambulance services, and initiated copwatch and armed self-defense against the police."[34] And then there is the Tubman Collective, which is organized by Black deaf and disabled activists. The Tubman Collective places disability justice squarely in the center of the Movement 4 Black Lives; members, too, conjure Tubman, who herself was disabled from a head injury caused by an overseer, in their effort to devise healing outside the prison and medical industrial complexes.[35]

Shira Hassan heralds liberatory harm reduction as a branch of healing justice. Hassan reminds us of the radical roots of harm reduction to challenge dominant approaches that rely on government funding and whitewashed ideals of health.[36] As she states, "The truth is that harm reduction was designed and created by drug users, sex workers, feminists, trans activists, people with chronic illness and disabilities, those of us working to end violence without the police, and those of us working to end prisons and the violent state. It is a practice steeped in joy, in living into the beauty of our lives no matter how messy they may (appear to) be."[37] Instead of pathologizing people who use drugs through a focus on "risky" use, liberatory harm reduction "emphasizes complete bodily autonomy" unencumbered from an ethos of free-market individualism.[38] It holds that people are not meant to be "fixed" into a whitewashed ideal and "honors the ways in which people live, survive, and resist oppression and violence by centering self-determination and by supporting people to be where they are."[39] Simultaneously, liberatory harm reduction aims to disrupt the sources of harm in the first place. In turn, proponents "envision a world without racism, capitalism, patriarchy, misogyny, ableism, transphobia, policing, surveillance, and other systems of violence."[40] Liberatory harm reduction, indeed, is *abolitionist harm reduction*.

A key point of healing justice, as Woodland states, is to recognize our intervulnerability to create "collective strategies for grief, joy, and celebration."[41] Indeed, through healing justice, grief can be channeled in ways that are oriented toward collective care and mobilization, as opposed to substantiating public officials' calls for vengeance, for instance, against people who deal drugs.[42] As Cindy Milstein writes in *Rebellious Mourning*, "Our grief—our feelings, as words or actions, images or practices—can open up cracks in the wall of the system. It can also pry open spaces of contestation and reconstruction, intervulnerability and strength, empathy and solidarity. It can discomfort the stories told from above that would have us believe we aren't human or deserving of life-affirming lives—or for that matter, life-affirming deaths."[43] In *Grieving*, Cristina Rivera Garza reminds us, when reflecting on the tremendous violence produced by the Mexican army and cartels, that suffering, pain, and grief produce connection: "Here, you and me, you and them, we together, we are in pain. We grieve. Grieving breaks us apart, indeed, and keeps us together."[44] To be sure, fostering a sense of communal grief requires an expansion of grievability not just for people who have over-dosed, which is already so important, but for all those who have been harmed by racial capitalism.[45] In doing so, as Garza continues, we can "radically revis[e] and alter[] the world we share."[46]

As is perhaps apparent, abolition is more than addressing individual social issues with individual clear-cut solutions. It is, as Ruth Wilson Gilmore states, "deliberately everything-ist; it's about the entirety of human environmental relations."[47] As such, the opioid crisis is not a singular social problem, nor is it solely about opioids, addiction, or overdose: It is about state violence, organized abandonment, neoliberal policy making, and the ongoing drug war within racial capitalism, which encompasses medico-carceral approaches that generate (treatable) carceral subjects in (therapeutic) carceral spaces, rooted in slavery and colonialism. Given the breadth of interlocking issues, abolitionists do not offer "one uniform vision" but "a range of approaches to work toward a liberated future."[48] Solutions are, as Kaba asserts, "built through struggle" and are particularly predicated on the experiences of those who are most marginalized and minoritized.[49] As Mari Matsuda puts it, "Justice means children with full bellies sleeping in warm beds under clean sheets. Justice means no lynchings, no rapes. Justice means access to a livelihood. It means control over one's own body. These kinds of concrete and substantive visions of justice flow naturally from the experience of oppression."[50] As capitalism is, and always has been, global in dimension, struggle exceeds national borders. Collective movement against state violence, as Derecka Purnell reminds us, is in constant motion, from Ferguson to Gaza and the West Bank.[51]

Inspired by abolition—of tearing down and building up—I end this book with a collection of local actions I deem as abolitionist care. Even if not formally labeled as such, they nevertheless reimagined and enacted "care beyond carceral logics of surveillance, punishment, and abandonment."[52] Actions included advocates and activists engaging in protest and daily mutual aid practices: of driving people to treatment and locating beds outside the criminal legal system, monitoring police stops, conducting jail visits and peer-led reentry support, and working to decarcerate and disinvest in jails and the larger criminal punishment apparatus. Some included rigorous planning, and others operated as forms of everyday, *ordinary* abolition, as necessary to resist violence-made-ordinary within racial capitalism.[53] Of note, I do not provide a granular analysis, nor do I consider the myriad of debates, conflicts, *and* failures that follow in movement building, across and within local and statewide organizing. Movements are certainly not frozen in fieldwork time, nor are organizers. Nevertheless, these actions offer a snapshot of local abolitionist imagining *and* doing—particularly in a time of opioid crisis. They thus encompass some of the "million different little experiments" that Mariame Kaba recommends for abolitionist organizing.[54]

Abolitionist Moments: "They're All Connected"

One way I arrived at this research was when attending a community-led protest at the Broome County legislature in 2014. Attendees were fighting against jail expansion. They held up signs reading, "NO TO JAIL EXPANSION" and "STOP JAIL EXPANSION." Despite community efforts, the expansion passed. This was a pivotal moment for the creation of the local grassroots organization Justice and Unity for the Southern Tier (JUST), which comprised a number of organizers and criminal-justice-impacted community members. JUST worked to decarcerate and disinvest from the jail while recommending, as cofounder Bill Martin has pressed, "funds for community-based and controlled health and education services that have been so severely cut by successive county administrations."[55]

JUST also held rallies at the jail, as well as at the hospital where the jail's privatized medical physician was employed. The group spearheaded a number of initiatives, including a jail visitation program to meet with requesting incarcerated people; Walk With Me, which provided peer-based reentry services; and Inside and Out, which held support meetings for family and friends of incarcerated people. JUST also networked with organizers across New York State. On December 1, 2017, members joined United Voices of Cortland (UVC) and Decarcerate Tompkins County (DTC) at the Cortland County legislature to stand in opposition to jail expansion, which would have cost the county $100 million, with $1.4 million already spent on the design of the jail. Protesters held signs that read, "NO more jails, not in Cortland, not in Broome, not in Tompkins counties." The Cortland County's Public Safety Needs and Assessment Committee declined to refer the expansion, and the primarily Republican legislature voted not to invest—it was a win.[56]

Yet, JUST's initial demands were also entrenched within the politics of health care and incarceration, or what James Kilgore refers to as "carceral humanism."[57] In a contribution to the activist-written anthology *The Jail Is Everywhere*, Andrew Pragacz and I wrote of how JUST's initial demands, which we helped create, were at times contradictory to the group's goals of divesting in the jail. JUST's 2017 action plan called for a reduction in incarceration and solitary confinement and an increase in judges' use of ROR (release on recognizance). Yet, the plan also proposed *improved* mental health resources with "proper funding," thus incorporating the rhetoric of building a "better jail" so often espoused by local officials.[58] As we documented the horrors of local incarceration in jail visits, letters, and lawsuits, this led to our stark conclusion: "Not one more dollar goes into this jail." Indeed, in 2018 Alexis Pleus, the founder and executive director of the harm-reduction nonprofit Truth Pharm, and I aired our concerns about state funding for privately operated treatment in the jail for the local *Press & Sun-Bulletin*: "A true win would be to offer MAT by a low-threshold, compassionate and trusted harm-reduction-based provider while putting a community oversight board in place to review all medical care at the jail. Simultaneously, efforts should be made to reduce incarceration rates, such as eliminating bail, while diverting funds to community services."[59]

Truth Pharm members also provided on-the-ground support for people who use drugs. Advocates searched for available treatment beds and offered transportation. When police threw out licenses that allowed people to possess needles, members wrote to the courts on their behalf. Truth Pharm held trainings on the use of Narcan, distributed fentanyl testing strips, and, for people coming out of jail, collected hygienic products and stored them in a local church. Advocates visited people in jail, held support spaces for those who lost loved ones to overdose, maintained that someone's recovery did not need to be abstinence based, and rebuked inpatient treatment restrictions such as bans on smoking cigarettes.[60] Members simultaneously marched and memorialized people who died from overdose at the local, state, and national levels, upholding harm-reduction and anti-incarceration principles. This work was empowering not just for family members but also for incarcerated and formerly incarcerated people. Interviewee Sarah, who was formerly incarcerated and worked with Truth Pharm, opted to wear Truth Pharm bracelets over where she had so long worn her jail identification bracelet, at least until she gets a watch, she added.

Local advocates and activists also highlighted the variety of needs people have beyond treatment support. Interviewee Mary, the peer-based reentry coordinator cited in chapter 5, spoke of the importance of addressing personal and structural factors for people coming out of jail: "You have to address the people as a whole, not sequentially, because there's the argument of, 'What comes first? Do you have to address their drug abuse or their mental health issues?' But they're all connected, so you have to do it together instead of sequentially, and you have to do it simultaneously. And reentry, substance use, mental health—it's all a part of it." The victim advocate Aaliyah, too, discussed in our interview the multitude of circumstances a person needs addressed before they seek treatment, including financial support, resources for children, and navigating abusive relationships.

Another local group, Progressive Leaders of Tomorrow (PLOT), organized "around issues of race, class, gender, and state violence through an anti-capitalist lens."[61] Aaliyah, who also worked with PLOT, stated that the group's focus was "especially for people that are marginalized, like people of color mainly, people with disabilities, people that are undocumented." In creating communal support, PLOT hosted a "Bystander Intervention Training" to provide methods to witness, record, and respond to police conduct, such as during police pedestrian stops. The group further promoted conflict resolution without calling police, taking a cue from "12 Things to Do Instead of Calling the Cops," jointly produced by the May Day Collective and Solidarity & Defense: "Sometimes people feel that calling the police is the only way to deal with problems. But we can build trusted networks of mutual aid that allow us to better resolve conflicts ourselves and move towards forms of transformative justice, while keeping police away from our neighborhoods."[62]

Aaliyah discussed how, as a victims advocate and member of PLOT, she at times had to switch between her advocate and activist hats when supporting people who had been harmed. Her advocate hat, as she put it, says, "'Report the crime to the police so that they can get the help that they need through the agency,' because you have to have a police report to get certain benefits." The activist hat, however, says, "Hell no, don't call the police," because you "don't want to cause any more harm to this person who already has bad experience with police." She offered the story of a Latinx woman she visited in the emergency room. As the woman did not live in the state, Aaliyah felt that filing a police report was unreasonable. So, she relied on mutual aid. As we ate at a Japanese restaurant, she recounted the situation:

> I asked her if she did a [police] report. She said the police told her to go to the hospital and call them from there. We called them from there. Then the police wanted her to go to the police station to file the report. And I'm like, "Well, she doesn't live—she has a black eye. She's kind of bruised up. She can't make it down there."
>
> So then she said that she didn't have anywhere to go. So it was suggested that she go to a shelter or something. She doesn't have any transportation, and she doesn't know her way around the community. So she said she would rather just take the bus and go home. So, I called the agency to see if they could have emergency funds to get a bus ticket for her. She would've had to leave the hospital, . . . go to the police station to file the report to get an emergency fund from the agency so she can be able to go home.
>
> . . . So she would have to go all the way to Endicott, get the police report, travel to Binghamton, go to the agency, get that. So I was like, "Oh no. This is a lot." . . . So I put the activist hat on. I contact PLOT, and I was like, "Listen, there's a woman of color here. She's stranded. She got assaulted, and she needs to get back to her family as soon as possible, and she lives [out of state]." So we get some funds to send her home. Stat. Got the funds. Went to buy the bus ticket. Gave her extra money for food while she was waiting for the ride, and she went home.

Collaboration across organizations, activists, and advocates was key to address interconnected forms of oppression. Truth Pharm coordinated with Pride and Joy Families, a group "dedicated to helping lesbian, gay, bisexual, transgender, and queer (LGBTQ) people in Upstate NY achieve their goals of building and sustaining healthy families."[63] During a public education event, the organizers discussed health-care impediments for LGBTQIA+ people, in turn challenging the heteronormative framing so common in local and national opioid reporting.[64] Collaborative direct action also occurred after three middle-school Black girls were strip-searched for drugs, because they appeared to school officials to be "hyper and giddy during their lunch hour." Activists filled a school board meeting in protest. Alexis Pleus sharply reminded in local reporting that "being 'hyper and giddy' are not common signs of substance use, and the district needs to be educated on signs and symptoms of drug use."[65] In a following protest, community members marched in front of the school on snow-filled streets. They held placards reading, "Happiness Among Black Girls Is Not a Crime" and "The AVG 12 y/o is 'Hyper and Giddy' STOP!! Shaming children of color!"[66]

Although I say "advocates" and "activists," it is more appropriately a collective "we." I marched, held signs, decorated varnished cardboard gravestones, and protested at county meetings, on the streets, in government halls, and at the jail. While there are certainly limitations to such engagement, as I discuss in the appendix, this approach brings about potential for abolitionist praxis.[67] After all, researchers are not detached observers but are immersed within the politics of meaning in which culture is made.[68] Thus, I aspired for a disruptive ethnography, a term developed with Andrew Pragacz, which is meant for researchers to intentionally enter the politics of meaning in the field for theoretical engagement and empirical investigation while advocating for and with those who are directly impacted.[69]

The connection between research and action was evident at Truth Pharm's 2017 Trail of Truth, a memorial event to commemorate the families of loved ones who died from overdose. Prior to the event, Pragacz, Pleus, and I compared opioid obituaries and jail release data to identify cases of individuals commemorated who fatally overdosed within two weeks of being released from the facility.[70] Pleus announced our findings at the event. As I wrote in my field notes, "On top of the stage at the plaza, adjacent to the downtown Binghamton main street, Alexis reports, 'Of the loved ones [commemorated], almost half had been incarcerated, and several memorialized died shortly after leaving the jail.' A woman in the crowd yells, 'That's my son!' before leaving in tears to be comforted by other attendees. A witness tells me later that the faces of the public officials sitting onstage were red the whole time."[71] In this research-action, we publicly highlighted the impact of reentry death, revealing to officials and attendees the afterlife of mass incarceration for those who died shortly after being released from the jail. Through families, friends, advocates, and activist-researchers, their memories would live on.[72]

Unpolicing Pain

There is so much pain in this research. Much is in this text. Even more is left in my notes, transcripts, and memories. I met so many people in pain; many were loved ones of those who overdosed or were incarcerated; many were parents who lost children and were left bereaved and angry. Many had been incarcerated and had overdosed, and some have since died. But the pain documented here is centuries old. It is at least colonial in origin, of Indigenous peoples hunted and scalped; of Africans shipped in chains and whipped into servitude; and of prison bars, chain gangs, and broken freedom. I wrote of Salladin Barton's death in the jail, with a correctional officer stating, "I'm a kill you N****r, I'm a kill you n***a," and of Makyyla Holland, who was misgendered, strip-searched, and beat up by correctional officers. There is Ronald Richardson, who was tragically killed by Jennifer Grenchus, who struggled with her own drug use. Formerly incarcerated interviewees spoke of being placed in solitary confinement, humiliated, hit on, and Ron told of being strapped to a restraint chair for days. Interviewee Niya relayed that she had been told to "go back to Brooklyn" more than she could count, and mug shots of Black people on the sheriff's Facebook page produced collective ire—of weaponized, retributive pain that only makes for mutual destruction.

As someone who has not lost a family member or close friend to overdose and who cannot imagine the direct pains of anti-Black racism—and sits on the white settler side of colonialism—the pain I interpret inevitably does not do justice to the complex lives that have felt it. It is curated pain, organized, placed on the page, and projected out, although it certainly commingles with my own pain, loss, grief, and struggles. It should be emphasized, then, that a catalogue of pain does not unpolice it. Indeed, without an abolitionist- and healing-justice-driven approach, pain research becomes a record of human suffering—with no meaningful intervention in sight. I must write, *we must write*, of pain, of their pain, of my pain, of your pain, of *our pain*, with intention: to unpolice it. To do so, we need to look to pain's roots in racial capitalism—for a pain made collective and mobilized.[73]

When thinking of a jailbreak of the imagination, I am reminded of interviewee Nate's recommendation of a center for dreamers: "I would make a center for different, different dreams, like dreamers and stuff, because addicts are dreamers; addicts are, like, gifted people. I think addicts are very misunderstood people that were almost insecure their whole life, because they knew they had a gift type of thing, and they were just numbing it because they didn't know how to utilize it. . . . I would have it go towards a center for dream building." In *Becoming Abolitionists*, Derecka Purnell also envisions a dream center for an abolitionist future. Inspired by Robin D. G. Kelley's account of Black struggle in *Freedom Dreams*, she states, "Our freedom dreams are the greatest threat to capitalism, colonialism, and the carceral state."[74] In this, communal pain must be paired with communal dream making—born out of collective resistance against racial capitalism.

I opened and closed this book with Laura's story, which represented a mixture of medicalization and criminalization in a time of opioid crisis. Her story was also a drug war narrative, as she entered a web of police, courts, and corrections for addiction recovery, with the carceral state being rendered a benevolent force, filled with caring cops, courts, and cages. And, as the drug war continues, whether through opioids or another substance (crack cocaine, meth, Xylazine), the terrain of policing and incarceration shifts and expands. To truly address the opioid overdose crisis, we cannot depend on carceral solutions. Rather, we need to cultivate abolitionist care to work against racial capitalism and its entailing racial policing. Unpoliced pain, indeed, is pain made revolutionary.

ACKNOWLEDGMENTS

There are so many people—indeed too many for this space—to acknowledge. I would like to start with those on the ground floor, including Juanita Díaz-Cotto, Gladys Jiménez-Muñoz, Travis Linnemann, Bill Martin, Aja Martinez, Joshua Price, Leo Wilton, and the Decarceration Working Group, John Eason, Luis Gonzalez, Brenden McQuade, Chungse Jung, and Andrew Pragacz. I would like to add a special recognition to Toivo Asheeke, Zoe Davis-Chanin, Jacqueline Frazer, Gabreélla Friday, Rae Jereza, Zhana Kurti, Cory Martin, Sung Hee Ru, Odie Santiago, Jordan Scott, and Hannah Walter, as our conversations and shared research interests proved essential for this work. I also have to give a shout-out to Frances Beal Society for keeping my mind and body in movement.

I would like to thank the folks in the Sociology, Anthropology, and Criminal Justice Department at Arcadia University, Jon Church, Ana María García, Doreen Loury, Favian Martín, Alex Otieno, and Dina Pinsky, as well as Margo Maas for her inspiring presentation for my Drugs & Society class. My gratitude also goes to Logan Fields for our ongoing conversations about drugs, addiction, and the drug war. Also, I must thank the Center for Antiracist Scholarship, Advocacy, and Action (CASAA), in particular Executive Director Christopher Varlack and Associate Director Favian Martín. I appreciate all the support I have gotten at SUNY Cortland, with special mention to Elizabeth Bittel. I would also like to acknowledge Stephen Philion at St. Cloud State University (SCSU) and Scott Foster at the St. Cloud Technical and Community College (SCTCC) for sparking my interest in sociology.

I offer special recognition to Alexis Pleus, the founder and executive director of Truth Pharm, as well as advocates including (but definitely not limited to) Shelley Canini, Corky Clark, Amy Cruz, Ralph DeRigo, Sam Hollenbeck, Jenni Horan, Susie Link, Jessica Saeman, Diane Semo, Christine Spivey, Kathy Staples, and, of course, Mitch. Rozann Greco,

Jackie and Denise Card, and Tina Gunther have also been an essential source of inspiration, as well as everyone in Justice and Unity for the Southern Tier (JUST). Without all of these people, this book would not have been possible.

I want to send my love to friends and family, including Doug and Carol Revier, Amy, Benny, and Indigo Bonnema, and Mike Champa for our drives. They have inspired me long before this research. I want to offer a special appreciation to Olivia Consol for being a constant source of encouragement—and for keeping me distracted during long days of writing. I would like to recognize students who have challenged and inspired me throughout the years. These include Marlie Ford, Lexi Kling, and Oli Lord. Students, truly, make this work worthwhile. Appreciation also goes to everyone who makes the New York University Press Alternative Criminology Series possible, with special attention to Jeff Ferrell, Ilene Kalish, and the helpful reviewers and editors.

Finally, I want to recognize those who have died from incarceration, policing, and overdose and those who are fighting conditions of oppression. And I would like to recognize those who have passed away, during and after my fieldwork, including Irene Difenderfer Aylward, Dominic "Dom" Davy, Benita Roth, Ty Tumminia, and interviewees who have since died from overdose and are not listed here by name. They lift us up as we fight.

Disruptive Ethnography and the Politics of Meaning

"Lock them up!" "Lock them up!" protestors yell in front of the head-quarters of Purdue Pharma in Stamford, Connecticut. They are calling out the Sackler family and Purdue executives for their aggressive marketing of OxyContin. Parents carry signs displaying names and photos of their lost loved ones. A father holds a placard with a picture of his daughter on a hospital bed; it is a jarring display. Artistic pill bottles scatter the sidewalk; they portray the skull-and-crossbones symbol next to text that reads, "SIDE EFFECT: DEATH." Posters stand upright on the sidewalk, one including a Photoshopped image of a Purdue Pharma executive behind prison bars. We advocates march in unison, carrying cardboard tombstones brought from New York. Protestors lie on the sidewalk, and others draw body outlines around them with chalk to depict a crime scene. After about an hour, the lead organizer provides closing remarks. He thanks the bordering police for being "here with us." The crowd disperses, leaving the chalk marks and pill bottles for passersby to bear witness.[1]

This excerpt reveals a variety of dimensions of what has been commonly referred to as the opioid crisis—of pharmaceutical industry (mis)conduct; of grieving, angry, and organized family members, friends, advocates, and people who use drugs and people in recovery; of police presence; of reporter coverage; and of a researcher conducting fieldwork, all surrounded by a theatrical display of pill bottles, posters, and tombstones atop a city sidewalk.[2] It is one of the many stages on which social problems, like the opioid crisis, play out.

It is evident then that social problems are not simply "out there" but must be identified as such. The social constructionist perspective, as Joel Best defines, considers how "people assign meaning to the world."[3]

The people who assign meaning to social problems are "claims-makers" who "say and do things to persuade audiences that a social problem is at hand."[4] Claims-makers include police, politicians, advocates, activists, reporters, researchers, scientists, and community members. In appealing to the public, claims-makers tell social problem formula stories, which produce "typical" representations of the social problem and of social groups, such as of greedy pharmaceutical heads or violent fentanyl dealers.[5] Winning claims-makers gain "ownership" over the problem, their narrative frames becoming the dominant, collective way of thinking about—and not thinking about—a social issue.[6] As David Altheide points out, "Frames focus on what will be discussed, how it will be discussed, and above all, how it will *not be discussed*."[7]

Social problem work operates within dominant ideology. Ideology is "the pervasive set of ideas that reproduce structures of dominance."[8] Within racial capitalism, dominant ideology is grounded on individual liberalism conducive for free-market exchange in land, labor, and commodities, all geared for capitalist profitability. Free-market individualism is associated with white freedom and order, which has required slavery as its contrast. As I quoted Saidiya Hartman in the introduction, "The slave is the object or the ground that makes possible the existence of the bourgeois subject and, by negation or contradistinction, defines liberty, citizenship, and the enclosures of the social body."[9] The social problem categories of "opioid user" and "drug dealer" are therefore steeped with racialized meanings surrounding white freedom and racialized enslavement and monstrosity, which drive police power to manage perceived drug-induced social disorder.

Police fabricate capitalist order by managing social movements and marginalized populations by employing the state's monopoly of violence. Broadly, the state "consists of the means of violence (the police and armed forces) in a given territory, together with state-funded bureaucracies (the civil service, legal, welfare, and educational institutions)."[10] It should be noted that the state is not merely an instrument of the capitalist class. Rather, it is a relatively autonomous sociohistorical product.[11] The capitalist state, in particular, is organized through class struggle.[12] Given the dominance of the capitalist class, state actors do cater to capitalist interests.[13] Generally, the capitalist state protects the liberty of contract, which, to varying degrees, facilitates exploitation, domination, and marginalization, all atop occupied land.[14] Police protect private property owners, and generally speaking, people are unable to call police on corporate actors.[15] Thus, within capitalist order, state power largely protects market freedom and private property for capitalist profitability.

Individuals are, consequently, *interpellated* as subjects of the state.[16] Interpellation occurs at the point of contact with state authority. When a police officer yells to someone walking down the street, "Hey, you there!," whether the person complies, runs, or fights, they are nevertheless rendered as subjects of state authority.[17] As Travis Linnemann puts it in *Meth Wars*, "The act of interpellation or becoming a subject of state power . . . occurs at the moment one responds to or recognizes state authority. . . . [This is a] dynamic political and cultural process of habitual subjection—in which individuals reaffirm their subordination to state power and authority."[18] In turn, state power operates through *pacification*, which involves coercion and consent.[19]

To be sure, there is persistent resistance to the labeling process. Meaning, as Stuart Hall argues, is "always challenged, contested, and transformed."[20] Consider the social problem category of the "meth user," as a degraded poor white figure. In Stacey McKenna's interviews with women who use meth, interviewee Bridget contrasted her consumption with the dehumanizing portrayals of meth users in The Meth Project campaign: "I just wanna know, do they just take a picture of somebody who's using meth or is that enhanced? 'Cause that right there would tell me. Come on, that's not fair, that's not right, that's false advertising."[21] Some people who use meth may maintain a positive self-image but by reinforcing stigmatized representations. Interviewees in Heith Copes and colleagues' research, for instance, established boundaries between their meth use and that of the "tweakers."[22] Jody Miller and colleagues found that women interviewees who use meth challenged dominant representations of the meth user but appealed to gendered standards of proper motherhood and beauty, as they spoke of the drug as helping them to maintain a clean house or lose weight.[23] Thus, people have agency to interpret meaning in creative, dynamic, and complex ways.

Overall, social problem work involves an interplay of cultural practices, related to claims-making, social problem framing, ideology, police power, interpellation, and resistance. Social problem categories like "user," "dealer," "addiction," "substance use disorder," "police," "recovery," and "treatment" thus contain raced, classed, and gendered meaning. Exploring how social problem making operates in the drug war therefore requires delving into the politics of meaning, where social problem making occurs.[24]

METHODS

When researching the opioid crisis in the Southern Tier region of New York from 2017 to 2019, I collected several forms of research documentation, derived from community meetings, interviews, media reporting, government files, personal journaling, and advocacy work.

I attended over eighty public meetings, such as, for instance, weekly meetings at the Broome County Opioid Awareness Council (BOAC), which was attended by the district attorney, county executive, sheriff, emergency services, and treatment and prevention specialists. I went to county legislature meetings, community forums, and public education events that involved local treatment specialists, affected family members, policy makers, and police. I observed drug court sessions and perused official documents, including the drug court and jail handbooks, county and city budgets, public meeting minutes, and state task force reports.

I conducted forty-four interviews, including with people who used drugs or were in recovery for drugs, family members of loved ones impacted by opioids, formerly incarcerated people, advocates and activists, harm-reduction specialists, prevention specialists, a county coroner, the county's emergency medical services (EMS) coordinator, and the Department of Social Services/Mental Health commissioner. To gather interviews and to get a scope of advocacy in the area, I first reached out to the local harm-reduction nonprofit Truth Pharm. I interviewed numerous members, including people who use or used drugs, family members of people who use or used drugs, and people in recovery. Interviewees provided names for other potentially interested parties, and the founder and executive director Alexis Pleus graciously posted my interest in interviewing people who use or used drugs on Facebook early in my research. I reached out to public officials online and during public meetings, and I collected contacts at public events and through my work with the local organization Justice and Unity for the Southern Tier (JUST).

I held interviews in coffee shops, restaurants, residences, diners, public offices, the public library, and Binghamton University's downtown center. Interviews were open-ended and averaged roughly an hour, ranging from thirty minutes to over two hours. I asked questions regarding how the interviewees defined the opioid crisis, experiences related to the crisis, treatment and criminal justice efforts in the county to address the crisis (referencing police, drug court, jail, treatment programs, and harm-reduction providers), and potential solutions. Regarding solutions, I asked, "If you had a grant with an infinite amount of money to address the opioid crisis, what would you do with it?" Of note, people who use drugs are largely viewed as untrustworthy. Yet, I had no reason to believe interviewees were lying about their experiences, especially given that the information was confidential. As Anne M. Fletcher summarizes the psychologists Mark Sobell and Linda Sobell,

> The bottom line is that if people believe what they are telling you will be confidential—particularly that it will not incur adverse consequences—and they are asked in a clinical or research context, then what they say tends to be reliable and valid. (This holds if the person has no substances in their system at the time of the inquiry.) But people are not stupid—if telling the truth about using drugs or drinking to a significant other, probation officer, schoolteacher, or work supervisor is going to bring trouble, why not lie and avoid the negative consequences? In short, if people have no reason to lie to you, the evidence suggests they will be truthful.[25]

It is worth noting that since interviewees knew that I was open to their experiences and had a stake in local advocacy, they may have also felt comfortable sharing. Alternatively, it may be argued that some told me what they thought I expected to hear, whether that meant praising or criticizing local actors and programs.[26] In addition, I did not identify as an opioid user or as someone in recovery, and I had not been incarcerated. As I grew up in Minnesota and was living in the area for graduate school, I was also somewhat of an outsider in the community. My interactions were certainly shaped by my status as a white, cisgender man, particularly when interviewing participants of color who discussed their experiences of harm in the community.[27]

Beyond formal interviews, I had many conversations when living in the area. If I mentioned my research at a local bar or when getting a haircut, residents at times discussed their personal use, familial use, and thoughts on the county's approach to the crisis. I interacted with reporters, correctional officers, police, attorneys, and a variety of public officials when observing court sessions or attending educational forums. I also communicated with interviewees before and after sessions. After my interview with Greg, he and I attended a Narcan training, and he eagerly updated me on the latest research in psilocybin treatment. I kept up with participants, often on Facebook, and for the few who did not show up for our interview, we still chatted, at times extensively, before scheduling.[28]

I also explored themes regarding the opioid crisis in local media.[29] This included, most prominently, *The Press & Sun-Bulletin*.[30] I accessed the reporting from an online database and retrieved microfilm for select articles, particularly to capture newspaper formatting and photographic display.[31] I read *The Ithaca Times* and kept up with local coverage by the news networks WBNG, Fox 40 WICZ TV, and NewsChannel 34 WIVT/WBGH. I considered social media, including advocacy groups' and public officials' Facebook pages. The sheriff's page, for instance, reported drug arrests and posted mug-shot photos. I considered the intended purpose, or "the marks of intent," of the material, such as of the sheriff's page presumably attempting to present a positive image of police and a negative one of the people arrested.[32] I analyzed popular reporting, such as Sam Quinones's 2015 *Dreamland* and 2021 *Least of Us* and Beth Macy's 2018 *Dopesick* and 2022 *Raising Lazarus*. Such writing constitutes a popular nonfiction opioid-crisis genre, which has influenced national and local conversations about opioids, addiction, policing, and overdose. Indeed, while I was unable to attend, a local church hosted a "community discussion" on Quinones's *Dreamland*. Members gave out copies of the book and advertised, "Everyone is invited to join us in reading this award-winning treatment of the subject."

I took account of everyday cultural documents. I snapped pictures of billboards citing treatment information or warning of drugged driving; of a bumper sticker informing that the driver has Narcan; and of an advertisement on a city bus reading, "Fentanyl is deadly and may be in your drugs." I saw commercials, such as one advertising a local syringe-service program that I watched on the waiting-room television at the jail; collected pamphlets in a local church citing "Signs &

Symptoms of Opioid Abuse"; and took note of a prescription drug drop box at the public library. I thus heeded Jeff Ferrell and colleagues' call for an interrogation of the everyday.[33] Billboards, commercials, brochures, and drop boxes thus act, as Mike Presdee put it, as the "debris of everyday life."[34]

Much of my engagement was advocacy and activist focused. I attended over seventy events and advocacy/activist meetings, and I worked closely with the local groups Truth Pharm and JUST. I participated in meetings (often taking meeting minutes), protests, memorial marches, opioid reversal trainings, and fundraisers (including a golf, psychic reading, and "free hugs" mall event), and I helped table events (such as for a local blues festival and community light festival called LUMA). I wore shirts with names of those who had overdosed; carried cardboard tombstones for family members unable to attend protests (a mother conveyed gratitude to me for carrying a picture of her son when marching); helped make tombstones as a form of protest and commemoration; laid down on pavement to get traced for body chalk outlines (and I traced others, too); participated in advocacy-led "die-ins"; attended memorial events; snapped pictures, for instance, of a balloon release on a warm summer day; and felt a sense of loss when finding out that an interviewee had passed away from overdose, adding to the grim reality of overdose death. I cowrote opinion articles, presented at local forums and conferences, and was interviewed by reporters.[35]

In such observation and action, I aspired for a disruptive ethnography, which occurs when the researcher intentionally enters into the politics of meaning in the field for rich theoretical engagement and empirical investigation while advocating for and with those who are impacted.[36] Indeed, disruption is a key concept in sociological research. Erving Goffman points out that "impressions fostered in everyday performances are subject to disruption," and ethnomethodologists have disrupted taken-for-granted norms to reveal social pressure in everyday life.[37] To be sure, fieldwork is inherently disruptive. Yet, intentionally disrupting state actors' claims, such as in a protest, produces movement-generated theory.[38] Disruption provides a crucial analytic: How will officials respond? What discourses will be mobilized? How can we push further?[39] Disruptive ethnography thus supports social justice goals while yielding insight on mechanisms of social control. In any case, such engagement felt unavoidable. In reviewing interview transcripts, I noticed a passage where I told advocate Stephanie of my inability to sit back and observe during meetings. As I told her, "When I started [research], I was just going to take notes, but then I realized I had to be in it. . . . I mean, I can go to a meeting and sit there, but if things are happening, if events are happening, I can't just be in the background totally."

Participating in local activism shaped my field engagement in key ways. For instance, I attended a local Copwatch event presented by Progressive Leaders of Tomorrow (PLOT), as I review in the conclusion. Inspired, I began to observe police stops, at times video recording and other times just sticking around. When walking home from the university's downtown center, I witnessed three young white men handcuffed and sitting on the sidewalk while police searched their vehicle. I stayed nearby to monitor the situation. The officers left, and one of the three men walked toward where I was standing. I asked if he needed help. He informed me that he just got out of rehab and was on probation. His friend had asked for a ride from a notable "hot spot" area that police regularly surveilled, and they pulled over the three. The friend had "stuffed" heroin in the backseat and was arrested with the other travelers. I offered contact information for Truth Pharm and asked if he needed further support. We then went our separate ways.[40] The police stop thus acted as a site of community intervention and advocacy, all while in the context of fieldwork.[41]

As another example, I went with Truth Pharm members to an educational event at a public school. Here, the county emergency medical technician (EMT) offered a variety of myths about fentanyl, which I analyze in chapter 2. At first, I acted as a passive observer, documenting the information provided by the speaker. My field notes turned into a field report. After the event, attendees and I shared the misinformation presented with fellow advocates, particularly regarding fentanyl as well as cannabis, as the EMT speculated that there had been a rise in overdoses in Colorado from cannabis legalization. Alexis Pleus and I emailed the county opioid prevention coordinator, challenging his claims.[42] The coordinator recognized our concerns and, as per our request, invited us to sit on the panel at the next event. Sitting with a police officer, a treatment provider, and the county executive, we publicly criticized policing and incarceration in the community.[43]

Such an approach was not without complications: It could be uneasy moving between researcher, friend, and fellow advocate and activist. At county meetings, I was at times an observer, a public commenter, or a protestor, shifting in ways that might always undermine another position.[44] My interviewee sample was not random, and advocate interviewees happened to be quite critical of local officials, although they certainly did not share a monolithic point of view. There is also a persistent concern I have of penal spectatorship, of participating in state-sanctioned voyeurism, such as when I observed interactions between participants and the judge in drug court.[45] As Saidiya Hartman reminds us of slavery's violence, and which is informative for carceral violence, we cannot "linger in scenes of slavery's violence without attending to the reproduction of the injury or the ethics of witnessing and the limits of empathy."[46] Importantly, this research was not designed through a participatory action framework, which, I believe, is ideal—if not necessary—for truly disruptive research. This writing is, thus, limited to much of my own interpretations, of course, informed by interviewees, advocates, and a wealth of critical writers. Nevertheless, I hope it adheres to an abolitionist praxis by challenging dominant opioid discourses that reinforce state power and by calling for and participating in collective action.

As a final form of documentation, I kept a field diary, which amassed over two hundred entries.[47] While originally intended to log interviews, schedule events, and reflect on field note observations, it became a place to emotionally process. I began to write about my own complicated relationship with drugs, alcohol, and sobriety. While I had not been a regular opioid user, I had heavily consumed alcohol, cannabis, nootropics, and at times kratom and some "harder" drugs (cocaine, MDMA, psilocybin). I considered positive experiences of drug use: of going out for beer after an advocacy meeting; of smoking cannabis with an interviewee in his living room; or of drinking whiskey and playing music with advocates on a porch, creating community in a cool summer breeze.

Yet, I recognized in my field diary that my drug use had been fueling anxiety and depression. At a particularly low point, I wrote, "And I feel like drinking and drugs is making things so much worse. Like I am comprised of somewhat disconnected parts, and smoking and drinking temporarily holds them together. Yet, when I'm hungover it's all ruptured and jagged, and flat. And what I've been repressing and the larger poisons of the drugs just sit in me, they are on my body. And I feel bloated, and fat, and tired, and ugly, and sick. This is like the first 10 pm I've been sober in, I'm sure, a long time."[48] Indeed, my ambivalence toward drug use led to various connections with interviewees, even if unbeknownst to them. This included when Paul described having an "addictive personality" or when Megan simply recognized the daily ups and downs of drug use. Shortly after leaving the field, I decided to quit for the long term. All this is to say that I have had my own embodied—and complicated—relationship with drugs, addiction, and sobriety in and out of the field.

Ultimately, my fieldwork was immersive, exploratory, and social justice oriented. Such an approach, I believe, is imperative to critically engage with the politics of drug use, addiction, treatment, pain, and the drug war, both locally and more broadly.

NOTES

INTRODUCTION

1 Author's field notes, 2019.
2 Lopez 2019.
3 Garnett and Miniño 2024.
4 CDC 2018; CDC 2023. In 2017, approximately two-thirds of fatal overdoses (47,600) involved an opioid (Wilson 2020).
5 Jacobs 2016; Leas 2017; Del Real 2017.
6 White House Council of Economic Advisors 2019.
7 White House 2016, 2018; ONDCP 2013.
8 BOP, n.d.
9 White House 2022b.
10 New York's opioid overdose death rate has remained steadily above the national average. From 2010 and 2021, opioid overdose deaths in New York rose from 12.3 per 100,000 residents to 32.7 per 100,000. Nationally, the death rate grew from 7.8 per 100,000 residents to 29.5 per 100,000 (NYS Comptroller 2022).
11 Reinhart, n.d.; NYS Senate, n.d.
12 Pragacz 2016; Subramanian et al. 2018. In 2023, there were 129,000 people incarcerated in jail on any given day. Eighty-four percent (109,000) were unconvicted (PPI 2024).
13 As Victoria Law (2021, vii–viii) defines it, "'The criminal justice system' refers to the legal system in which people are arrested, prosecuted, and threatened with imprisonment." Rather than provide justice, however, the system "metes out punishment." This has caused many people to adopt the terms "criminal legal system," "criminal processing system," and "criminal punishment system." To be sure, the term "criminal" is not to be taken for granted, given that many who are processed through the system have not been convicted of a crime, criminal courts process criminal charges and not "criminals," and what is labeled a "crime" and who is thought of as a "criminal" are political.
14 Native Land Digital, n.d.
15 Aswad and Meredith 2001, 14.
16 Zahavi 1988, 22; Town of Binghamton, New York, n.d.
17 O'Donovan 2014, 290.
18 O'Donovan 2014, 291.

19 O'Donovan 2014, 287.

20 O'Donovan 2014, 287.

21 O'Donovan 2014, 289.

22 Shay 2012; Bing, n.d. The city's population doubled between 1880 and 1890 (Seward 1924; Rubin 2016, 15).

23 IBM began as the Bundy Time Recorder Company in downtown Binghamton (Aswad and Meredith 2005).

24 Britannica Money 2024.

25 O'Donovan 2014, 275–276.

26 Pragacz and Revier 2024, 78.

27 The university also spread to the urban core with a university annex building, a privately developed student housing complex, and a pharmacy in Johnson City (O'Donovan 2019, 285). Through the state-sponsored granting program Restore NY, Binghamton received $7.59 million over three years to demolish or rehabilitate residential and commercial properties with "shovel ready" lots for private development (O'Donovan 2014, 294–295).

28 Developers and corporations have tended to take advantage of tax benefits before leaving (O'Donovan 2019, 295).

29 Barnes 2021; NYS Comptroller 2024; World Population Review, n.d. The Binghamton racial composition in 2023 was white (non-Hispanic), 82.8 percent; Black or African American (non-Hispanic), 4.95 percent; Asian (non-Hispanic), 4.42 percent; two+ (non-Hispanic), 3.17 percent; and white (Hispanic), 1.87 percent (DATA USA, n.d.).

As a note on the population decline, 16,776 residents left between 1970 and 2010, from 64,123 to 47,347 (Census Reporter 2021). Unemployment was 5 percent in 1990, 10 percent in the early to mid-2010s, and 17.5 percent during the COVID-19 pandemic; it returned to 5 percent in 2023 (Bureau of Labor Statistics 2023; Abel and Deitz 2019). Yet, the number of employed residents dropped by one-fifth, from one hundred thousand in 1990 to eighty thousand in 2022 (Bureau of Labor Statistics 2023).

30 Shay 2012, ix–x.

31 In this regard, Broome County suits what Jack Norton et al. (2024b, 1) refer to as a nationwide "quiet jail boom."

32 Pragacz and Revier 2024, 79; Norton et al. 2024b.

33 Bureau of Labor Statistics 2023. As David Harvey (2017, 22) points out of state and punishment-generated revenue, "The state can become a driving force in accumulation to the degree that it exercises powerful influences over effective demand for military equipment, police and surveillance technologies, and a variety of instruments of social control."

34 Broome County, n.d.-a.

35 In regard to the total operating budget, from 2013 to 2023 the District Attorney's Office funds rose from 0.68 percent to 0.97 percent of the budget. The Probation Office increased from 0.70 percent to 0.93 percent. The Public Defender's Office

dropped from 0.55 percent to 0.53 percent. The Sheriff's Office budget went from 8.53 percent to 9.94 percent (Broome County, n.d.-a).

36 City of Binghamton, n.d.

37 NYS DOH 2018. In 2016, there were seventy-six fatal overdoses. Reports of fatal overdoses per year are as follows: sixty-six in 2017, thirty-two in 2018, thirty-seven in 2019, thirty-nine in 2020, fifty-four in 2021, eighty in 2022, sixty-seven in 2023, and forty-eight in 2024 (BOAC 2024).

In 2016, the overdose death rate "involving any opioids" in Broome County was 29.3 per 100,000, only to be outdone by Erie County (29.8 per 100,000) and Ulster County (30.2 per 100,000). By 2021, it was 37.7 per 100,000, behind Chautauqua County (37.9 per 100,000), Sullivan County (46.4 per 100,000), Greene County (47.4 per 100,000), and Bronx County (48.3 per 100,000) (NYS DOH 2024b).

38 Roby 2015.

39 Broome County 2017, 30.

40 Broome County, n.d.-a; Broome County 2017, 189.

41 Broome County, n.d.-a.

42 Broome County, n.d.-a.

43 Whyte 2014.

44 Cavender and Fishman 1998. There are numerous issues with the dominant representation of police. Most crimes are not reported to police, and police do not solve many of those reported to them (Statista 2024a). The crimes police interact with on a daily basis are not the violent felonies so often depicted in the media (Vitale 2017). Indeed, a study of New Orleans, Montgomery County (Maryland), and Sacramento found that 4 percent or less of the calls to police were for violent offenses (Asher and Horwitz 2020). The theory that police deter crime is largely unsubstantiated (Boivin and de Melo 2023), and the Supreme Court has deemed police as not having a constitutional duty to protect the public (*Town of Castle Rock v. Gonzalez*, 545 U.S. 748 [2005]). Furthermore, corporate crime, which is not well monitored, perpetuates more public harm than does "street crime" (Kappeler and Potter 2017).

45 Neocleous 2021, 2.

46 Wood 2017, 2.

47 Thier 2020, 7.

48 Vitale 2017, 34.

49 As Viviane Saleh-Hanna (2015) states of Black feminist hauntology, "Through this lens the modern day police officer is haunted by, developed by, *born out of* his original self—the slave catcher."

50 Thier 2020, 13.

51 Thier 2020, 15.

52 Thier 2020, 18; Marx (1867) 1990, 896–897. Of note, this legislation appears to have never been put into practice. Nevertheless, it represents "the widespread vilification of the poor" (Isenberg 2016, 22).

53 Isenberg 2016, 28.

54 Federici 2004, 27.

55 Not private property but *security*, Karl Marx (1844) reminds us, is "the highest social concept of civil society" (Neocleous 2021, 8).

56 Karl Marx ([1867] 1990, 925) wrote of the connection between wage labor in Europe and slave labor abroad, "While the cotton industry introduced child-slavery into England, in the United States it gave the impulse for the transformation of the earlier, more or less patriarchal slavery into a system of commercial exploitation. In fact, the veiled slavery of the wage-laborers in Europe needed the unqualified slavery of the New World as its pedestal." See Thier 2020, 21–22.

57 Kendi 2016.

58 ASHP, n.d. Boston, Philadelphia, and New York were the center of international slave commerce (Manjapra 2022, 11–12). William Bingham owned enslaved people (Martin 2022c), and Joshua Whitney Jr. was the first person to bring "Negro slaves into Binghamton" to work in his $4,000 mansion (Aswad and Meredith 2001, 15).

59 Hadden 2003; Dunbar-Ortiz 2018, 70; Vitale 2017, 46.

60 Vitale 2017, 46–47. The 1661 and 1688 slave codes in the British Caribbean colony of Barbados, as Roxanne Dunbar-Ortiz (2018, 40) reviews, "extended the task of controlling enslaved Africans from overseers and slavers to all white settlers, in effect shifting private responsibility to the public."

61 See Kelly Hayes's (2022) interview with Ruth Wilson Gilmore.

62 Owens 2022, 164.

63 Hartman 2022, 258. Rubio-Ramos 2022, 3.

64 Novak 2014, 4.

65 Rubio-Ramos 2022, 3.

66 Curtin 1992; Blackmon 2009. As Angela Davis (2003, 29) puts it, "Vagrancy was coded as a black crime, one punishable by incarceration and forced labor, sometimes on the very plantations that previously had thrived on slave labor."

67 K. Williams 2023, 59. Consider the case of the Floridian freedwoman Hannah Tutson. White men invaded her home and separated her from her husband and three children, and she was "beaten and repeatedly sexually assaulted by the deputy sheriff" (K. Williams 2023, 128–129).

68 Equal Justice Initiative (EJI) documents over four thousand people killed by vigilantes between 1877 and 1950 (Stevenson 2017, 13; EJI 2017). R. Gilmore 2007, 178; Davis 2003; Purnell 2021.

69 Churchill 2004.

70 Dunbar-Ortiz 2018, 41.

71 Dunbar-Ortiz 2018, 45–46.

72 Isenberg 2016, 34–35.

73 Razack 2020, 2.

74 Dunbar-Ortiz 2018, 37.

75 Dunbar-Ortiz 2018, 36.

76 Vitale 2017, 43.

77 Vitale 2017, 41.

78 Vitale 2017, 41. In Binghamton, a nonunionized cigar workers' strike over a wage dispute in 1890 was ended after three and a half months when local police arrested participants on the picket line (O'Donovan 2014, 288).

79 As Julian Go (2020, 1196) states of the nineteenth-century professionalization of the police, it was a way "to penetrate civil society with a legitimacy that militaristic forces lack."

80 Neocleous 2014.

81 In this regard, racism is not merely individual prejudice but a system of meaning that symbolically and materially benefits those who are labeled as white (Tatum 2017).

82 Haney-López 2006. In *Dred Scott v. Sandford* (60 U.S. 393 [1857]), Chief Justice Roger Taney reasoned in the majority opinion of the denial of citizenship for Black people, "They had for more than a century before been regarded as beings of an inferior order, and altogether unfit to associate with the white race, either in social or political relations; and so far inferior, that they had no rights which the white man was bound to respect; and that the negro might justly and lawfully be reduced to slavery for his benefit" (Powell 2022, 216).

83 See Kendi 2016, 7.

84 Hartman 2022, 342.

85 The race scientist and French aristocrat Arthur de Gobineau (1915, 205) wrote that in his three-part system, "the negroid variety is the lowest, and it stands at the foot of the ladder" (Strings 2019, 149). Indeed, Blackness would act as a marker to demarcate presumably degraded whites. Gobineau (1915, 74), for instance, described southern and eastern people as inferior "hybrid" whites, indicating, as Sabrina Strings (2019, 149–150) explains, "that although they are not as degraded as Africans, they were nevertheless 'only civilized on the surface.'" One anthropologist explained that the "predominant mouth of some Jews" was "the result of the presence of black blood" (Kendi 2016, 295).

86 Hartman 2022, 342. Indeed, the 1661 Virginia Act designated slave status specifically for Africans, which replaced reliance on white indentured labor. Such laws were instrumental in suppressing cross-racial movement, such as with Bacon's Rebellion (1676–1677). It is important to consider, too, how the system of chattel slavery developed from indentured labor and, thus, the class system in England. Nancy Isenberg (2016, 42) documents "three interrelated phenomena": "harsh labor conditions, the treatment of indentures as commodities, and, most of all, the deliberate choice to breed children so that they should become an exploitable pool of workers."

87 Hartman 2022, 104.

88 Robinson 2020; Wall 2020. This image is largely based on Thomas Hobbes's ([1651] 1982) *Leviathan*, in which he recommends a sovereign body to prevent a "war against all" within the state of nature.

89 Micol Seigel (2018, 12) adopts the term "violence work" to describe policing: "The essence of police work extends, therefore, beyond the patrol or the service call

and far beyond the uniformed, public police to the much larger category of people who do violence work. People authorized to inflict violence might be ratified by a nonstate agent such as a private company, or be part of a mob enjoying effective social sanction, as with the KKK or other lynch mobs. Either way, such people are also channels for violence condoned by the state."

90 Purnell 2021, 5–6.

91 Wall 2016.

92 Hart 2021; NIAAA 2024.

93 In 2019, around 2.6 million deaths were considered to be alcohol related world-wide (WHO 2024). The World Health Organization (WHO) estimates that tobacco "kills more than 8 million people each year" (WHO 2023b).

94 Becker (1963) 2008.

95 Taylor 2016.

96 The Harrison Act mandated the purchase of stamps for import, manufacture, and distribution of opium or coca and their derivatives. For people in possession without "a written prescription issued by a physician, dentist, or veterinary surgeon," penalties included fines up to $2,000 and five years of imprisonment (Caquet 2022, 164; Musto 1999). The act had global influence. Three US delegates, most prominently Hamilton Wright, pushed for international drug prohibition at the First International Opium Commission of 1909, which was attended by thirteen nations in Shanghai. As P. E. Caquet (2022, 150) puts it, "The ideas that intoxicants were something to be managed rather than combated, that their non-medical use might be acceptable under certain circumstances, or that addiction might more easily and usefully be treated than stamped out all died in Shanghai."

97 Caquet 2022, 128–129.

98 Knipe 1995.

99 *New York Times* 1908; Caquet 2022, 125. The opening of China to the opium trade was a result of the Opium Wars between China and Great Britain (1839–1842, 1856–1860). This influenced Chinese opium smoking, which spread from the wealthy to the workers. The opium den subsequently "became the symbol of the drug's ubiquitous progress" (Caquet 2022, 75–78). And still, opium use in China was not at the level of public perception. There were approximately fifteen million regular smokers, which represented 3.3 percent of the population. While "a far from negligible level," P. E. Caquet (2022, 78) concludes, "it is nowhere near impressionistic notions of an entire country held in drug slavery."

100 Cobbe 1985; Hickman 2000, 73.

101 *Medical and Surgical Reporter* 1887, 684; Caquet 2022, 125.

102 Hickman 2000, 77.

103 This was despite Black Americans being unlikely to use cocaine, in part due to economic disadvantage (Caquet 2022).

104 E. Williams 1914; Fisher 2022, 128.

105 Nolan 2001, 24.

106 Police departments upgraded from .32 caliber bullets to the .38 Special cartridge, which became "the standard cartridge of most police departments for decades to come." Fisher 2022, 129; Wells (1892) 2013; Feimster 2022.

107 Rush 1784. Rush identified several aspects of alcoholism: that it is progressive, that it produces a loss of self-control, and that abstinence is the only cure. In contrast, during the seventeenth and most of the eighteenth centuries, habitual drunkenness in colonial America was considered a moral choice; it was a sin but not a disease-like compulsion (Levine 1978, 47).

108 Levine 1978, 45. The disease concept of addiction developed after the end of prohibition, particularly from the self-help organization Alcoholics Anonymous, the Yale Research Center, and the work of E. Morton Jellinek (1960; see Schneider 1978). Importantly, this work placed the source of addiction within the diseased individual rather than the drink, thus moving addiction from the bottle to the body (Levine 1978).

109 Gusfield 1986. An 1871 political cartoon by Thomas Nast portrayed an Irishman holding a bottle of liquor while sitting on a gunpowder keg that reads, "Uncle Sam." The cartoon is titled "The Usual Way of Doing Things" (Walfred 2016).

110 *Binghamton Press*, September 9, 1925; see Rubin 2016, 20. Binghamton was the largest municipality to vote itself dry. Prior to national prohibition, as Jay Rubin (2016, 19) documents, "in an outpouring of wartime fervor and religious zeal, city residents voted overwhelmingly to close saloons and outlaw the sale of alcohol."

111 Rubin 2016, 20. As Jay Rubin observes, while the 1923–1928 organizing efforts by the KKK in Binghamton were largely unsuccessful, the politics of prohibition and policing nevertheless linked logics of white supremacy and nativism with extrajudicial and judicial state violence.

112 Hari 2015.

113 Anslinger and Cooper 1937; Hart 2021, 161.

114 Solomon 2020; Vakharia 2024, 24; Szalavitz 2016, 26.

115 Caquet 2022, 221.

116 *New York Times* 1927.

117 Caquet 2022.

118 The Boggs Act mandated minimum sentencing that ranged from two to ten years for drug violations, with longer sentences for repeat offenses. The Narcotic Control Act mandated "five to ten years for the first offense and ten to forty years without the opportunity for parole for the second, and a maximum of life in prison or the death penalty for providing narcotics to a minor" (Caquet 2022, 233).

119 Lassiter 2023, 185.

120 Ehrlichman continued by stating, "[By] criminalizing both heavily, we could disrupt those communities, arrest their leaders, raid their homes, break up their meetings, and vilify them night after night on the evening news. Did we know we were lying about the drugs? Of course we did" (Baum 2016). These efforts quelled

midcentury social movements and heralded the neoliberal turn toward law-and-order policy (R. Gilmore 2007).

121 See Bradford 2021.

122 Courtwright 2010.

123 Washton 1986, 58–59; Reinarman and Levine 2004, 185; Fisher 2022, 88. Scholars refer to such designations as "pharmacological determinism," in which drugs appear to be "endowed with uniquely addictive or 'enslaving' powers strong enough to determine human behavior" (Fisher 2022, 81). Yet, 70 percent or more of people who use drugs do not meet the criteria of a substance use disorder; this includes for heroin and methamphetamine (Hart 2021, 11).

124 UPI 1982; see Forman 2022, 351.

125 Zakaria 2012; PPI, 2024. Nearly half of the federal prison population is imprisoned for a drug crime (BOP 2024).

126 Mancuso 2010, 1536.

127 Campbell 2010.

128 Rush 1812. As Harry Levine (1978, 52) explains, with moral treatment, "the mad could be freed from their chains and taught to constrain themselves."

129 National Park Service 2017.

130 Schneider 1978; Wilkerson 1966.

131 Caquet 2022, 344–345. Narco thus acted as a prison, therapeutic community, and clinical research center (Campbell 2010).

132 Jerome Jaffe devised "a drug-budget formula where far more funds (70 percent) went to treatment than to incarceration (30 percent)" (Macy 2022, 84; Massing 1998). New York Governor Nelson Rockefeller also embraced methadone programming before signing the punitive Rockefeller drug laws in the 1973 (Kohler-Hausmann 2010, 76).

133 DOJ 1986. The 1994 act allocated "$383 million for prison drug treatment programs, including $270 million in formula grants for states" (DOJ 1996).

134 Kaczynski 2019.

135 As Brenden McQuade (2020, 66) reminds us, "public education, penology, social welfare policies, and public health are all administrative projects that continually reproduce capitalist social relations."

136 Dammer and Albanese 2013, 99.

137 As the slave owner Thomas Jefferson argued, "despotism produced disease, democracy liberated health" (Porter 1999, 57; Sullivan and Ballantyne 2023, 18).

138 Hartman 2022, 291; Cable 1907. The French anthropologist and naturalist Julien-Joseph Virey claimed in his 1837 *Natural History of the Negro Race* that Black people were, as paraphrased by Sabrina Strings (2019, 85–86), "mindless, self-gratifying automatons who were 'given up to the pleasures of the table, those great eaters, intemperate epicures who seem to live only to eat, have a stupid look. . . . Always digesting, they become incapable of thinking.'" Similarly, in *The Inequality of the Human Races*, Arthur de Gobineau (1915, 205) contended of the gluttonous nature of Black people, "The very strength of his sensations is the most striking

proof of his inferiority. All food is good in his eyes, nothing disgusts or repels him. What he desires is to eat, to eat furiously and to excess" (Strings 2019, 149).

139 As Hartman (2022, 280) puts it, "The linking of whiteness with purity, neatness, morality and health accedes to a politics of contagion that eventually serves to justify segregation and license the racist strategies of the state in securing the health of the social body."

140 Fatsis and Lamb 2022, 49. Mark Neocleous (2003, 5) points out that imaginings of the state through metaphors, such as the body politic, are "ways of making us think about and orient ourselves to the state and the kind of order it is engaged in producing." In turn, "members of civil society come to *imagine* themselves through the categories which the state has generated for their administration" (2003, 60).

141 Indeed, fascist states often combine political and medical discourse, such as when promoting "racial hygiene" (Neocleous 2003, 30). David Courtwright (2019, 98) observes the connection between temperance, policing, and nation-building; as he points out, "By the 1930s hygienic policing was a hallmark of all modern states, and an obsession of fascist ones." A German addiction authority in 1938 contended, for instance, that "citizens did not have the right to destroy their bodies with poisons" and that "the belief that 'your body belongs to you' was Jewish Marxist claptrap." As Courtwright continues, "Real Real Germans bore the torch of Teutonic ancestry. They kept their bodies fit for their clan and people. Alcoholics who thought otherwise risked sterilization, the fate of perhaps thirty thousand heavy drinkers, mostly lower-class men. Others wound up in the camps" (99).

142 Loseke 2003, 28.

143 Loseke 2003, 40.

144 Loseke 2003, 17.

145 Consider that when participants in a 1995 study were asked, "Would you close your eyes for a second, envision a drug user, and describe that person to me?," 95 percent identified an African American man or woman (Burston et al. 1995, 20).

146 Wray 2006.

147 The British doctor Sir Williams Collins (1915) recognized in a lecture that drug prohibition contradicted the "sanctity of individual choice." Yet, he reassured that "alcohol and drug addiction are to be regarded as examples of the surrender of self-control in favour of self-indulgence." It follows that, as P. E. Caquet (2022, 152) paraphrases Collins's logic, "one should not be allowed to surrender one's own liberty voluntarily." Thus governmental intervention, to Collins (1915), appeared justifiable: "It is the restraint of liberty to secure a larger and truer liberty."

148 Ingraham 2014; Hamilton Project 2016; Rosenberg et al. 2017.

149 Beckett 2022.

150 Greer and Jewkes 2005, 21.

151 For information on interviews, see the appendix.

152 The concept of addiction has been used to describe the excesses of drug war policing. Marc Krupanski (2017) wrote for *Stat News*, "It's time to kick our addiction

to the war on drugs." California Deputy Attorney General Gary Shons also used the metaphor of addiction to describe police's reliance on asset forfeiture: "Much like a drug addict becomes addicted to drugs, law enforcement agencies have become dependent on asset forfeitures. They have to have it" (Ehlers 1999, 3).

153 Garriot 2011; Reinarman 2005. Of note, addiction emerged as a legal category, not from medical discovery. As P. E. Caquet (2022, 279) reviews, "Drug prohibition had not been constructed from a scientific consensus, and even less so was it expanded, in the 1960s, based on more precise science. It was the other way around: the scientific consensus was made to fit the mission creep of expanding prohibition." As he continues, "While the terms changed, at heart remained the age-old question: did drugs make the user sufficiently unfree to justify his or her punishment or forcible confinement by the state?" (2022, 356).

154 Hartman 2022. The term "addiction" stems from the Latin word *addicere*, which means "given over to." It was used to describe how a debtor could be enslaved to a creditor. Carl Fisher (2022, 20) adds that *addicere* also referred "to a strong devotion or a habitual behavior" or a "strong preference." As I have argued, the term "addiction" within racial capitalism is connotative of Black enslavement as the counterpoint to white liberal freedom. For instance, the Quaker abolitionist Anthony Benezet (1778, 42) wrote, "The unhappy dram-drinkers are so absolutely bound in slavery to these infernal spirits, that they seem to have lost the power of delivering themselves from this worst of bondage." In 1774, the writer and planter Landon Carter linked the excessive gambler to the enslaved African: "These are fellows which talk of freedom, but no African is so great a Slave, as such are [they] to their Passion for gaming" (J. Greene 1987; Courtwright 2019, 85).

155 Dubber 2000. As Robin Room (2003, 226) puts it well, "Addiction can be seen as a secularized and rationalized form of ideas about possession, which had traditionally been thought of in terms of usurpation of a person's being by an alien spirit, something which entered the afflicted person from the outside and took control of the person's behavior against his or her will." Thus, as Desmond Manderson (2005, 35) observes, "The crime of possession is the sin of being possessed." Indeed, fears of white racial possession are long-standing, with the Black devil possessing Puritans into witchcraft (Kendi 2016; Gagnon 2021) or Black Voodoo practitioners manipulating whites in dance and ritual (Long 2007).

156 As Sabrina Strings (2019, 6) states of the anti-Black underpinnings of fat phobia, concerns about body weight are not about health but "have been one way the body has been used to craft and legitimate race, sex, and class hierarchies." Du Bois (1903) 2015.

157 Beletsky and Davis 2017; Binswanger et al. 2007; Merrall et al. 2010; Lim et al. 2012; Ranapurwala et al. 2018; Degenhardt et al. 2014.

158 Metzl 2024.

159 R. Gilmore 2024, xii. The drug war, then, can be understood as a literal war "fought on the terrain of class relations" (Linnemann 2016, 223). James Baldwin,

for instance, deemed the Anti-Drug Abuse Act of 1986 as a "bad law" that would "only be used against the poor" (CSPAN 1986; Hart 2021, 28).

160 Hayes and Kaba 2023.

161 Arani 2022, 13.

162 I elaborate on disruptive ethnography in the appendix.

163 Neoliberalism is, broadly defined, a political-economic formation that includes the deregulation of corporations; the privatization of public goods; the gutting of the social safety net; the attack on labor; the exploitation of low-wage, precarious, flexible, and part-time employment; consumption through incurring debt; and reliance on incarceration and policing for economic investment and to regulate inequality and crises (Thier 2020; Harvey 2007, 2). Frydl 2021; Herzberg 2021.

164 Sack 2018.

165 Penn 2019.

166 Biviano 2018.

167 Johann Hari stated in an interview with *British GQ* (Schofield 2024), "And I'm very concerned that there could be an opioid crisis-like death toll from young girls—and it is overwhelming young girls—and boys starving themselves."

168 Reinarman 1994, 92; Jenkins 1994.

169 Linnemann and Medley 2023, 430.

170 Sullivan and Ballantyne 2023. Of note, the American Pain Foundation, which "described itself as the nation's largest organization for pain patients," received 90 percent of its $5 million of funding in 2010 from the drug and medical-device industry, according to a ProPublica investigation (Ornstein and Weber 2012).

171 Chiarello 2024. Travis Linnemann and Corina Medley (2023, 419) utilize the term "palliative capitalism" to refer to "a set of social relations in which legal pharmaceutical drugs and their producers, marketers and distributors profit from treating or attempting to treat the conditions that capitalism creates."

172 Sykes (1952) 2007. Punishment within the criminal legal system, as Nils Christie (2007, 5) reminds us, "means the inflicting of pain, intended as pain." Indeed, the terms "pain" and "penality" derive from the same Latin root.

173 B. Alexander 2010.

174 Statista 2024b.

CHAPTER 1. MEDICALIZING OUR WAY OUT OF THIS

1 CDC 2017a; BOAC 2017; author's field notes, December 2017.

2 Between 1991 and 2005, opioid prescriptions more than doubled in the US, from 76 million to 163 million (Volkow 2014). Overdose deaths nearly tripled within thirteen years, from fewer than 10,000 in 1991 to 29,800 in 2005 (Katz and Katz 2018; Lupick 2022, 30). The prescribing rate is prominently due to Purdue Pharmaceutical's marketing of OxyContin in 1996. The Food and Drug Administration (FDA) approved OxyContin for moderate pain, and the company promised twelve-hour pain relief with little chance of addiction. It assured that "only 1% of takers become addicted" when citing a four-sentence letter to the editor in the

New England Journal of Medicine (Porter and Jick 1980). Nearly seven hundred sales reps marketed to approximately one hundred thousand physicians, many in suburban, small-town, and rural areas. Purdue offered physicians vacations, gifts, and ongoing medical education (Hansen et al. 2023b, 146). From 1997 to 2001, OxyContin distribution increased tenfold for non-cancer-related pain (Van Zee 2009). Purdue generated more than $35 billion from OxyContin sales (US House of Representatives, Committee on Oversight and Reform 2021).

3 Revier 2020a.

4 Hazlitt 2016.

5 ABC News 2010; Schwartz 2012; Lee 2013; Leas 2017; Amsden 2014; Helling and Flemming 2017; Netherland and Hansen 2016.

6 The white overdose rate in particular has been linked to health-care access and doctor prescribing patterns (Herb et al. 2021). OxyContin was originally marketed for "trustworthy" and "legitimate" patients coded as white (Hansen et al. 2023a, 39). Black pain has also been perceived as less serious by medical providers, as based on the stereotype that "Blacks are impervious to pain" (Washington 2022, 207; Meghani et al. 2012; Wyatt 2013; Singhal et al. 2016).

7 Richards 1981. Black fatal overdose rates have also increased markedly from fentanyl (Bechteler and Kane-Willis 2017; James and Jordan 2018; Case and Deaton 2020). Furthermore, non-Hispanic Native Hawaiian or other Pacific Islander (NHOPI) and non-Hispanic American Indian and Alaska Native (AIAN) people "experienced the largest percentage increases in drug overdose death rates from 2020 through 2021, with rates increasing 47% (13.7 to 20.1 per 100,000) and 33% (42.5 to 56.6 per 100,000), respectively" (Spencer et al. 2022, 3).

8 Bechteler and Kane-Willis 2017. The focus on prescription opioids also over-reports the connection between painkiller prescription, addiction, and overdose (Muhuri et al. 2013; SAMHSA 2015).

9 Seelye 2015; see Beckett and Brydolf-Horwitz 2020.

10 Cobbe 1985; Hickman 2000, 73.

11 Hansen et al. 2023a, 37; G. Bush 1990.

12 ONDCP 2013.

13 Volkow and Collins 2017. Numerous medical institutions have provided information on the opioid crisis, including NIDA's "Opioid Overdose Crisis" (2019); the NIH's "Health Research and Development to Stem the Opioid Crisis" (2018); the Centers for Disease Control's "Understanding the Epidemic" (2017b); and the World Health Organization's (WHO's) "Opioid Overdose" (2023a).

14 Netherland 2023.

15 As Philip Athans (2014, 31) writes, "We find that a lot of our archetypical and famous monsters are transformed people: vampires, werewolves, mummies, zombies, pod-people, *The Thing*, *The Fly*, and so on."

16 The "white addict" expresses what Noël Carroll (1990, 43) refers to as "ontological fusion," as they "transgress categorical distinctions such as inside/outside, living/dead, insect/human, flesh/machine, and so on" (D. Gilmore 2009, 9).

17 Author's field notes, June 2017.

18 I used the term "substance use disorder" when speaking to a reporter to describe the importance of proper medical care for incarcerated people (Perez 2019). For the benefits of harm-reduction initiatives, see research on MAT (Connery 2015; Wakeman et al. 2020), naloxone access (McClellan et al. 2018), syringe-service programs (Des Jarlais et al. 2005; Abdul-Quader et al. 2013), and supervised injection sites (also referred to as overdose prevention centers; Marshall et al. 2011; Lupick 2022). Of note, OnPoint NYC runs two overdose prevention centers in New York City, which have been shown to decrease overdose risk and public drug use (Harocopos et al. 2022).

19 PPI 2024. Catering to this population, in 2014 the Federal Bureau of Prisons (BOP) replaced the term "substance abuse disorder" with "substance use disorder" in order "to be in line with the DSM-5" (BOP 2014).

20 DeFulio et al. 2013.

21 Ultimately, for addiction to be medicalized, researchers must employ medical language, and medical intervention must be applied to "treat" the condition (Conrad 1992, 211). Drug researchers, in turn, produce a taken-for-granted collateral reality of addiction "as a particular kind of problem" (Moore and Fraser 2013, 922; J. Law 2009; Campbell 2007; Fraser et al. 2014). A "disease" thus "does not exist until we have agreed that it does—by perceiving, framing, and responding to it" (Rosenberg 1989, 1–2; Reinarman and Granfield 2014, 2).

22 Hart 2021, 8–9.

23 Hart 2013, 301.

24 NIDA 2007, 5.

25 Leshner 1997, 46; Fisher 2022, 64.

26 Volkow 2015 (emphasis in original); Fisher 2022, 64.

27 Medical research implies a white figure, as it relies on the seventy-kilogram white male (Hansen 2023, 21; see also Bonilla-Silva 2012). By appealing to a universal, deracialized subject, brain scans, as Helena Hansen and colleagues (2023a, 37) argue, "expunge the racial identity of the addict, . . . [leaving] a racially unmarked and thus implicitly white social figure."

28 As P. E. Caquet (2022, 362) adds, "In lay parlance, the idea of the 'hijacked brain' has taken the place of the nineteenth-century 'disease of the will.'" Indeed, the idea that drugs *hijack brains* (Volkow and Li 2005, 1430; *Harvard Mental Health Letter* 2011; Rodolico 2016; Sinha 2018) evokes Black criminal street crime against a symbolically white figure.

29 The *DSM* is used by psychiatrists and other mental health professions to diagnose mental illnesses. The 2013 *DSM-5* covers ten classes of drugs, including alcohol, hallucinogens, and opioids, with subset disorders, such as alcohol use disorder and opioid use disorder. SUD is measured on a continuum from mild to severe, with a mild substance use disorder requiring two to three symptoms from eleven criteria.

30 Room 2003, 226.

31 Keane 2002, 4.

32 Fraser et al. 2014, 43.

33 Quinones 2021, 144.

34 Quinones 2021, 5.

35 Neocleous 2016, 32, quoting Locke (1689) 1980, 11.

36 Hinton and Cook 2021.

37 Kendi 2016, 24 (emphasis added).

38 Kellogg 1907, 522; Strings 2019, 180 (emphasis added).

39 Ford and Revier 2023.

40 Stanciu 2021, 114.

41 Quinones 2021, 259. The zombie framing of drug use is clear in historical accounts of addiction. The 1928 bestseller *Dope: The Story of the Living Dead* (Black and Older 1928) "described drug addiction as 'a wasting, loathsome, hideous, cruel disease' and people with addictions as 'carriers' of a disease 'worse than smallpox, and more terrible than leprosy'" (summarized by Fisher 2022, 144). The magazine *Current Literature* (1889) further documented zombie-like transformation:

> The habit seems more a disease than a vice, for the whole nature of the victim undergoes a complete revolution, moral, mental, and physical. . . . The flesh begins to fall away and the space around the eye becomes dark from being surcharged with blood; the skin loses its normal color and changes to a sodden gray, a blotched brown, or an unhealthy yellow. And then the victim shivers and perspires at the same time, and is easily moved to tears. When this stage is reached there is little hope of a cure. They must and will have the drug, and will resort to any device to procure it. (quoted in Caquet 2022, 121)

42 Quinones 2021, 341.

43 Miles 2015, 43. bell hooks (1992, 168) writes that zombie-like behavior by enslaved people was a response to the condition of slavery: "Reduced to the machinery of bodily physical labor, black people learned to appear before whites as though they were zombies, cultivating the habit of casting the gaze downward so as not to appear uppity. To look directly was an assertion of subjectivity, equality. Safety resided in the pretense of invisibility." See Holland 2000, 15; Linnemann et al. 2014, 508.

44 Métraux 1959, 282. Thus, the zombie is "a form of Worker: a living dead slave-labour, an alienated person robbed of their will and controlled by a master-sorcerer" (Neocleous 2016, 48).

45 Neocleous 2016, 52. Philip Athans (2014, 24) points out that the monster "has the ability to hit closer to home, describing the human potential to become inhuman."

46 Quinones 2021, 5; Stanciu 2021, 112; Sheff 2013, xvi. The zombie, as Neocleous (2016, 60) writes, has become "increasingly understood in terms of the 'outbreak' of some kind of contagious disease, virus, or plague."

47 Sheff 2013, xvi. Or we can consider the demonological aspects of addiction discourse in Sheff's (2013, xi) phrasing that people become "*afflicted* with addiction." See Atrens 2000.

48 Daniels 2012. Addiction signals not just individual wasted whiteness but disruption of the white family. The white family is, as Frantz Fanon (1967, 127) puts it, "the educating and training ground for entry into society." Of further note, physical transformation can be a consequence not of drug use per se but of poverty and a lack of health care and harm-reduction services. Abscess growth, for instance, can result from unsanitized equipment. As Dr. Kim Sue told the journalist Travis Lupick (2022, 45), "when intravenous drug users have low-barrier and affordable access to sterile injection equipment, abscesses are rare and there is little chance of contracting HIV or any other virus." Abscess formation can also occur when missing a vein, which, too, can occur from a lack of education or from injecting in less-than-ideal circumstances, such as doing so surreptitiously in public spaces where police may be present. See Lupick 2022, 73–74.

In addition, people who use drugs regularly betray the "zombie" image by living "meaningful and even rewarding lives," as Edward Preble and John Casey (1969) found in their research on people who use heroin in New York City. The critical addiction scholars Craig Reinarman and Robert Granfield (2014, 9) make this point well: "Preble and Casey showed instead that so-called street addicts had to engage in a challenging round of activities every day in order to avoid being dope sick, and that, however illegal and destructive, their cycles of stealing, scores, and shooting often provided meaningful and even rewarding lives compared to the limited array of legal options available to them."

49 Room 2003, 229–230.

50 Wall 2020, 324. As Philip Jenkins (1999, 11) puts it, "The idea that drugs can reduce users to primitive savagery is inextricably bound up with the racial fears that have always been so critical an element of America's drug scares."

51 Neocleous 2016, 32. Medical metaphors thus "frame action possibilities" (Simon 2001, 1070). On drug-induced zombification and police violence, see Travis Linnemann et al. 2014.

52 Williamson 2016.

53 Murray 2012, 131; Confessore 2012; Pruitt 2019, 123. Moynihan (1965) reported, "In practically all its divergences, American Negro culture is . . . a distorted development, or a pathological conditions, of the general American culture." See Kendi 2016, 3.

54 Tunnell 2004. Consider degraded representations of people who use meth in the Faces of Meth campaign (Linnemann and Wall 2013; Linnemann 2016) or in Quinones's (2021, 259) description of meth as creating in West Virginia a drug-induced "caste of people." Indeed, the white poor of colonial America were viewed as producing a "new breed of human" (Isenberg 2016, 56).

55 Case and Deaton 2020.

56 Case and Deaton (2020, 2) deem the term "deaths of despair" a "convenient label": "We came to call them 'deaths of despair,' mostly as a convenient label for the three causes taken together. Exactly what kind of despair, whether eco-

nomic, social, or psychological, we did not know, and did not presume. But the label stuck, and this book is an in-depth exploration of that despair." Of further note, while the US spends much on health care, a lack of investment in public health infrastructure has subsequently created "the worst health outcomes of any industrialized nation" (Hansen et al. 2023a, 25). In addition, the US is the only wealthy country that does not have universal health care (Sullivan and Ballantyne 2023, 82).

57 The journalist Eric Eyre (2016) found, "Between 2007 and 2012, drug wholesalers shipped more than 780 million hydrocodone and oxycodone pills into [West Virginia]." This amounted to "433 pain pills for every man, woman and child in West Virginia." Overall, the US prescribes 80 percent of the world's opioids (Degenhardt et al. 2019; Sullivan and Ballantyne 2023, 48).

58 This situation is compounded by perceived white disadvantage compared to working-class African Americans (Case and Deaton 2020, 5). Despite a rise in white mortality rates, Case and Deaton (2020, 65) do recognize that "black mortality rates in 2017 were only slightly lower than those experienced by whites forty years earlier."

59 Case and Deaton 2020, 212.

60 Ruhm 2022.

61 Case and Deaton 2020, 2.

62 Friedman et al. (2023) point out that, between 1999 and 2013, the 9 percent documented increase in premature deaths among white people "did not come close to catching up to the mortality rate among Black Americans; . . . to reach parity, the rate would have had to increase by more than 50%." Furthermore, premature deaths of Native Americans increased by nearly 30 percent. In 2020, the rate was double that of white Americans. The authors refer to the lack of publicity as "data genocide."

63 Hansen 2023, 21.

64 bell hooks (2006, 169) has highlighted the importance of such cultural inquiry, writing, "When intellectuals, journalists, or politicians speak about nihilism and the despair of the underclass, they do not link those states to representations of poverty in the mass media."

65 M. Bell 2007.

66 Case and Deaton 2020, 28.

67 Quinones 2015, 4. In *Methland*, Nick Reding (2010) depicts a meth-induced binary in rural Iowa, writing, "Main Street was no longer divided between Leo's and the Do Drop Inn, or between the Perk and the Bakery: it was partitioned between the farmer and the Tweaker." Linnemann 2016, 150.

68 Linnemann 2016, 143.

69 Rebecca Scott (2010, 37) argues that generic representations of Appalachia merge people with topography: "Appalachian stereotypes conflate the land and people, with dark, trash-filled hollows sheltering isolated, incestuous communities." See Schept 2022, 24. Indeed, explorers, amateur scientists, and early ethnologists

professed of the colonial poor that "inferior or mismanaged lands bred inferior, ungovernable people" (Isenberg 2016, 56).

70 Weller 1965; Karshner 2019, 280. Weller (1965, 37) writes, "While tradition can thwart the planners and molders of industry, education, and society in general, fatalism can so stultify a people that passive resignation becomes the approved norm." Nancy Isenberg (2016, 137) further notes that nineteenth-century observers identified low-income whites as "ruin[ing] themselves through their dual addiction to alcohol and dirt."

71 Macy 2018, 42.

72 In reviewing mortality data, Christopher Ruhm (2022, 1183) points out that "rising overdose deaths probably primarily reflected a supply-driven phenomenon, with demand-side factors influencing who was most affected . . . only one of which was despair." This contrasts from Case and Deaton's demand-side argument that "opioids fueled the fire of existing despair." Indeed, Case and Deaton's use of despair is at times contradictory in the text. They describe it as a "convenient label," but it also appears to be "a deeply rooted indicator of great unhappiness" (Ruhm 2022, 1171).

73 Case and Deaton 2020, 39–40.

74 Case and Deaton 2020, 39. Case and Deaton (2020, 2) state that deaths of despair are "self-inflicted, quickly with a gun, more slowly and less certainly with drug addiction, and more slowly still through alcohol." They do recognize, in any case, that "many, even in the grip of their addiction, and even when they understand that they will die if they cannot break out, do not want to die" (2020, 96).

75 hooks 2006, 169.

76 Case and Deaton 2020, 95. They further adopt the language of slavery and carcerality in the rest of their explanation: "Addiction, it is often said, is a prison where the locks are on the inside, but that makes escape no easier. The 'selfish brain' cares only about ensuring that the habit gets fed, and it makes people unable to care about how they behave, the havoc they create, or the lives they destroy" (2020, 95).

77 Tunnell 2004, 135.

78 Author's field notes, March 2019.

79 Belenko and Spohn 2014, 59. Kenneth Tunnell (2004, 136) observed that the states with the highest per capita OxyContin use had *lower* property crime rates than those with the lowest per capita use. In Broome County, the property crime rate declined between 2013 and 2023, from 3,135.8 per 100,000 to 2,172.7 per 100,000 (NYS DCJS, n.d.). To be sure, some people do steal for funds to obtains drugs (Kuhns et al. 2012). The nonprofit Truth Pharm conducted a survey with a non-random sample of 190 respondents in the Southern Tier and found that, while awaiting treatment, 93 said they committed a crime to meet the needs of their addiction (Roby 2017). Nevertheless, the concerns of a *rise* in property crime can be overstated and, to be sure, mixes with larger media-generated fearmongering surrounding drugs, crime, and public safety.

80 Neocleous 2021, 117.

81 O'Donovan 2019, 274.
82 O'Donovan 2019, 290. George F. Johnson presented an image of a "warm friend-ship" between managers and workers inside and outside the factory. He referred to their mutual loyalty as the "Square Deal." Yet, he did not do so through a sense of benevolence but for labor discipline. He was antiunionist and favored competi-tive piece work. Factories had maggots and roaches, toxic output, injury-causing machines, hot temperatures, and women workers experienced sexual harassment (Shay 2012; O'Donovan 2014). It should be noted that workers did negotiate loy-alty by asserting their end of the "Square Deal" bargain. Instead of accepting wage reductions, as Gerald Zahavi (1988, 118–119) accounts, "workers might refuse cer-tain jobs if they felt they were poorly priced. They would join together to restrict output. They criticized and isolated fast workers whose pursuit of individual gain threatened the collective interests of coworkers. They loafed on the job, gambled, talked back to supervisors, refused to work on unpleasant jobs, engaged in acts of individual sabotage, or simply walked out of the factory, never to return, for any number of reasons."
83 Hansen 2023, 21; Schept 2022.
84 Isenberg 2016, xii.
85 Case and Deaton 2020, 6. The authors do contend that the 2016 election of Donald Trump would "make things worse, not better" (2020, 13). Nevertheless, as Ruhm (2022, 1184) writes, "Social conservatives will be happy to construe the myriad problems of less educated whites documented in *Deaths* as evidence of the need to return to traditional values, although that is not Case and Deaton's interpretation."
86 Linnemann 2016.
87 Beckett 2022. Of note, a focus on self-infliction in despair research downplays structural circumstances that drive overdose deaths, such as a lack of harm-reduction services and prohibition itself.
88 Talbot 2017.
89 Faces of Opioids, n.d.
90 Betty Ford Institute Consensus Panel 2007, 222 (emphasis added); SAMHSA 2016, 3. See also D. Frank 2018.
91 Cohen 2000, 598.
92 Beman 1829, 6–7 (emphasis added); Levine 1978, 49.
93 Room 2003.
94 As Suzanne Fraser and colleagues (2014, 58) put it, "The addicted individual is . . . realised as a target for particular forms of regulation and intervention in order to restore the idealised state of autonomy, control and productivity reified as normal [i.e., white] and healthy existence."
95 Campbell 2010, 94 (emphasis added).
96 Vrecko 2010, 45 (emphasis added).
97 Foucault 2010; Strings 2019, 7.
98 Lupick 2022, 218; Netherland 2023, 89.

 99 Frank et al. 2021; Hansen 2017.

100 Hansen et al. 2023a, 34.

101 A 2005 national study found that 91 percent of buprenorphine patients were white (Stanton et al. 2006), and a 2019 study found that "whites were still three to four times as likely as Blacks to receive buprenorphine, and the vast majority of those receiving buprenorphine (at a cost starting at $300 per month) paid for it with cash or with private insurance rather than Medicaid or Medicare" (Lagisetty et al. 2019; paraphrased by Hansen 2023, 11).

The whiteness of buprenorphine was apparent in the passing of the 2000 Drug Addiction Treatment Act (DATA), which permitted physicians to prescribe buprenorphine. Health and Human Services Director Donna Shalala stated that buprenorphine was meant for those "who would not normally be associated with the term addiction" (*Congressional Record* 2000, 19112; see Hansen et al. 2023a, 42). Advertisements for buprenorphine largely depicted white patients (Hansen et al. 2023a, 44).

102 Of note, the New York Department of Health (NYS DOH 2024a) best practices recognizes that "patients are typically more forthcoming with a complete report of substance use, when there are no punitive responses and no threat of discontinuation of care with an unexpected toxicology test result." See Jarvis et al. 2017.

103 Generally, one in ten people who seek treatment receive it (ASAM 2017). Treatment access is even scarcer in rural counties (AAMC 2017). The nonprofit Truth Pharm conducted a survey with a nonrandom sample of 190 respondents in the Southern Tier and found that participants "typically faced lengthy waits trying to access treatment. For half of them, more than two weeks passed between when they reached out for treatment and their first evaluation. After that, 75 percent waited at least a week before entering a treatment program. Only 8 percent entered within three days" (Roby 2017). Interviewee Michelle discussed the difficulty of receiving treatment for her son, Lucas: "They have to call every hour on the hour to try to get a bed, and it can literally take days for them to get a bed. And when an addict, you know, finally agrees to start calling, it's just literally days to get in."

104 As Kay stated in full, "I would honestly open up a rehab full of addicts that had gotten sober and wanted to fight to change the stigma, but make it a rehab where these mothers, who are single mothers, can have their children in there with them, also where the families could come and learn everything they need to know on how to do the steps to help their loved one change. There's nothing like that. You can't bring your kid with you to rehab. So that whole time, you're without your child. Your child's hurting 'cause they don't have you."

105 Author's field notes, May 2019.

106 Indeed, Kay's explanation fits NIDA's (2020) explanation of addiction: "The initial decision to take drugs is typically voluntary. But with continued use, a person's ability to exert self-control can become seriously impaired. This impairment in self-control is the hallmark of addiction."

107 Atrens 2000, 21; Revier 2022, 327.
108 Lembke 2021; Maté 2008, 142.
109 Carl Fisher (2022, 63–64) suspects that, while "even the most dyed-in-the-wool scientists don't actually mean to argue that" neuroscience is the only way to describe addiction, "the implication is there, and it does have consequences."
110 Seear and Fraser 2010, 440–441 (emphasis added). Indeed, medical explanations were employed to pathologize resistance by enslaved Black people. The term "dysaesthesia aethiopica" was used by doctors and scientists for enslaved people who "engaged in work stoppages, 'property' destruction, or 'theft'"; thoughts of escape were deemed "drapetomania" (Lewis 2021, 38).
111 Fisher 2022, 64. The temperance lecturer John B. Gough (1881, 433) described drunkenness as "a sin" but "also a disease," a "physical as well as moral evil" (Levine 1978, 49).
112 Link and Phelan 2001.
113 Hartman 2022, 8. As Hartman (2022, 8) states in full, "The value of blackness resided in this metaphorical aptitude, whether literally understood as the fungibility of the commodity or as the imaginative surface upon which the master and the nation came to understand themselves." In *Black Skin, White Masks*, Frantz Fanon (1967, 167) also drew on the ways in which Blackness serves the white imaginary; he observed, "In Europe the black man has a function: to represent shameful feelings, base instincts, and the dark side of the soul." The literary uses of what Toni Morrison (1993, 7) refers to as "American Africanism" furthermore "provides a way of contemplating chaos and civilization, desire and fear, and a mechanism for testing the problems and blessings of freedom."
114 Neocleous 2003, 24.

CHAPTER 2. THE DEALER DIVIDE
1 The billboard was funded with money seized from drug dealer arrests (Joseph 2016).
2 Beckett and Brydolf-Horwitz 2020.
3 Beckett 2022, 28; PDAPS 2019. Drug-induced-homicide laws are also referred to as "death by distribution" and "drug delivery resulting in death" laws. Since 2011, thirty-nine states and Washington, DC, passed legislation that increases penalties for drug crimes involving fentanyl (Collins and Vakharia 2020). Health In Justice (2020) found an increase in cases of drug-induced homicide from 495 in 2016 to 717 in 2017, and there was a 300 percent increase in reporting on such cases between 2011 and 2016, from 363 to 1,128 (DPA 2017; Beckett 2022; Beletsky 2019).
4 Borrelli 2016f.
5 Linnemann and Medley 2023, 416. As Richard Nixon commented of people who deal drugs when introducing the Comprehensive Drug Act to Congress (US Congress 1970), "However far the addict himself may fall, his offenses against himself and society do not compare with the inhumanity of those who make a living exploiting the weakness and desperation of their fellow men." See Herzberg 2021, 293.

6 Beckett 2022, 62.

7 D. Gilmore 2009, 1.

8 Newman 2017; Washington 2022, 205.

9 Delgado and Stefancic 1992.

10 Hamilton Project 2016; Ingraham 2014; Rosenberg et al. 2017. Seventy-five percent of cases of federal sentencing for fentanyl trafficking involved people of color (Collins and Vakharia 2020), and drug-induced homicide prosecutions are more often brought when the person who died is white (Beletsky 2019, 874). People of color have also received median sentences three years longer than those of whites (Goulka et al. 2021; Netherland 2023, 78–79).

11 By saying this, I do not mean to deracialize death. Rather, it is important to recognize ways in which racial capitalism kills whites. Consider, for instance, how the access to opioids for middle-class whites led to a heightened overdose rate (Hansen et al. 2023b) or how the politics of racial resentment, which has increased gun availability and gutted health care and education, has contributed to the white mortality rate (Metzl 2024). I thus stress here the anti-Black underpinnings of *white death*.

12 Billings 2017.

13 Herzberg 2023, 93.

14 Sullivan 2018; O'Brien 2013; Linnemann 2016. The novelty of suburban drug addiction is apparent in descriptions like "suburban junky" (J. Hassan 2012).

15 Reinarman and Duskin 1992; Lipsitz 2007; Lassiter 2023.

16 Borrelli 2017a; Whyte 2017.

17 Borrelli 2017f.

18 Broome County is part of the High Intensity Drug Trafficking Area (HIDTA), which provides police federal funding for "zone defense to drug trafficking," as Senator Chuck Schumer put it (Borrelli 2015b). To be sure, the mapping of "high intensity" areas produces insecurity through the imagining of widespread drug trafficking and "the promise of heightened policing intensity" (Linnemann 2016, 175).

19 Netherland and Hansen 2016, 659.

20 Netherland and Hansen 2016, 676.

21 Spectrum News Staff 2016.

22 *Binghamton Homepage* 2016a (emphasis added).

23 Russell 2018 (emphasis added).

24 Grondahl 2014, 27; Greer 2007. Her mother, Patty Farrell, was a retired police officer. When advocating for the law, Farrell utilized the user/dealer divide, as a reporter paraphrased: "She pleaded for expanded treatment for addicts, tougher penalties for dealers, increased investigations and heightened vigilance by overly trusting parents." See Wright 2016.

25 Madison 2019. Brindisi's comments were in support of the 2018 International Narcotics Trafficking Emergency Response by Detecting Incoming Contraband with Technology (INTERDICT) Act, which funded US Custom and Border Protection

personnel and scientists "to interpret data collected by such devices during all operational hours" (US Congress 2018).

26 Neocleous 2003, 109.

27 Lipsitz 2007, 12.

28 A photograph of the bumper sticker was shared with me by Jacqueline Frazer.

29 In the local newspaper, Alexis Pleus and I made the argument that uploading such mug shots by the sheriff's department promotes racial stereotypes about people who use and deal drugs, as many posted were people of color (Pleus and Revier 2017). We did, rather regrettably, use a "race neutral" framing of the opioid crisis when writing, "There is no 'us' and 'them,' no 'white' or 'black,' no 'dealer' or 'user,' there is simply an addiction epidemic that needs to be treated as a health care crisis."

30 E. Anderson 2015.

31 Mohamed and Fritsvold 2009.

32 Coomber 2006, 141.

33 J. Eaton 2017.

34 Macy 2018, 9.

35 Macy 2012a.

36 Borrelli 2017c. The other two were a Latinx man and a white woman. Both pled guilty. I did not find sentencing comments in local news reporting (see Borrelli 2016c, 2016d).

37 Borrelli 2017c.

38 Borrelli 2017f.

39 Borrelli 2017b.

40 Borrelli 2017c.

41 I am not claiming intentional racial bias by the court (Lawrence 1987). Sentencing relates to a myriad of factors, including statutes, criminal record, seriousness of conduct, and judicial discretion. Nevertheless, people of color are more likely to receive higher sentences, often related to "past criminal involvement" (Belenko and Spohn 2014, 190–191). As Steven Belenko and Cassia Spohn (2014, 213) further review, "Gender- and race-linked attributions of dangerousness, threat, and potential for reform continue to influence judges' evaluations of appropriate punishment for drug offenders."

42 Chancer 2010; Revier 2018.

43 Mills 1940.

44 See Ayres and Ancrum 2023. It should be noted that low-level drug dealing is not as lucrative as often perceived, as profits largely move to the top of the supply chain (Salinas 2023; Rios 2011). Indeed, many people who deal drugs still work part-time and full-time jobs, which Jeffrey Fagan and Richard B. Freeman (1999) refer to as "doubling up" (see Salinas 2023, 227). Far from deviating from societal norms, people who deal drugs can uphold neoliberal ideals of entrepreneurship, self-reliance, profiteering, competitiveness, and conspicuous consumption (Ayres and Treadwell 2023).

45 For interviewee Megan, an addiction to the lifestyle was not a proper motive to deal drugs: "I hate 'em [dealers]. . . . I mean, they made good money
off of me. . . . [They'll state,] 'I'm just doing it for my family.' 'No you're
not. . . . You're addicted just like we are. You're addicted to the lifestyle
I'm giving you.' . . . I look at drug dealing as like an addiction. . . . You can
be addicted to the money, you know, the fast money. . . . It's very different
[from drug addiction] but very similar at the same time."

46 R. Gilmore 2007, 178. As Sylvia Federici (2018, 55) has it, "Poverty resulting
from cuts in welfare, employment, and social services should itself be considered a form of violence, and so should inhumane working conditions."

47 Author's field notes, February 2019.

48 Public officials offered competing reasons for dealers cutting heroin with
fentanyl. A Monroe County public forum report by the Senate Task Force
(NYS Senate 2014) explained that adding fentanyl was not meant to kill
the person but to maintain a "long-term customer": "The drug dealers can
add fentanyl to the heroin as a booster and to make it more powerful. The
goal of any drug dealer is to make you a long-term customer. Once they
have you, they can quickly increase prices for it, knowing that you will
need the drug." Either way, this explanation and the EMT's both focus on
the intent of the individual dealer, not structural circumstances.

49 Interviewee Jim made this point about fentanyl awareness: "You fuck
yourself because you're like, oh, there's fentanyl dope in Johnson City.
You're fuckin' advertising it." See Reinarman and Levine 1997, 44; Brecher
1972.

50 Beletsky and Davis 2017.

51 Lupick 2022, 131–132.

52 Beletsky and Davis 2017.

53 Hart 2021. Indeed, people who deal drugs can be essential in providing a
safer drug supply. The executive director of the North Carolina Survivors
Union, Louise Vincent, offered an example in Travis Lupick's *Light Up the
Night* (2022). She purchased heroin that made her sick. She called the seller,
and he "returned promptly, apologized profusely, and gave them [her
and her fellow travelers] back their money. And he pulled the rest of that
batch off the street." He told her, "No way, I don't want to be responsible
for a death" (Lupick 2022, 191). Indeed, Vincent has helped people who
deal drugs maintain a safer supply. As she informed, "One guy, he trusts
me, and we're showing him dilution and how to cut and what to cut with.
And how to test for fentanyl. . . . You get them thinking in terms of money
and also in terms of not killing their customers" (Lupick 2022, 203–204). I
would like to make note of Vincent's (2022) broader criticism of Lupick's
writing.

54 DEA 2016. The DEA (2016) has also listed safer ways of handling fentanyl. On top
of this, the agency has warned of "rainbow fentanyl" (DEA 2022) and has referred

to fentanyl overdoses as poisonings, implying intent "by a nefarious and deceptive drug dealer" (DEA 2024; see Hampton 2024, 129).

55 Changing the Narrative, n.d.

56 Changing the Narrative, n.d.

57 P. Smith 2018. In *Overcoming Opioid Addiction*, the physician Adam Bisaga (2018, 30) describes fentanyl as an "ethereal weapon." Beth Macy (2018, 283) and Anthony King (2019, 254) further substantiate this myth in *Dopesick* and *Addiction Nation*, respectively.

58 For an overdose to occur, fentanyl must make direct contact with mucous membranes or in the bloodstream through snorting, smoking, or injection (O'Neill and Wheeler 2017).

59 Linnemann 2022, 155–156.

60 Borrelli and Murray 2017. In Henry Brownstein's (1991, 89) seminal work, he identifies New York City news coverage (from 1986 to 1990) of white pedestrians being caught in the crossfires of drug-related gang disputes. A *New York Times* article in his sample read, "Brutal Drug Gangs Wage War of Terror in Upper Manhattan."

61 Riback 2017. Between 2011 and 2017, the Attorney General's Organized Crime Task Force (OCTF) took "down 25 large drug trafficking gangs, made more than 580 felony narcotics arrests, and seized more than $1.5 million and more than 2,000 pounds of illegal drugs" (NYS OAG 2017).

62 In Broome County, the violent crime rate has fluctuated but overall increased between 2013 and 2023, from 259.2 per 100,000 to 280.8 per 100,000. Indeed, Broome County has had a higher violent crime rate in comparison to surrounding counties. The 2023 crime rate in adjacent counties was as follows: Chenango County (146.6 per 100,000), Cortland County (223.7 per 100,000), Delaware County (per 134.9 per 100,000), and Tioga County (111 per 100,000) (NYS DCJS, n.d.). Nevertheless, it is important to recognize that the *imagery* presented by journalists and politicians of widespread crime and gang violence tends to sensationalize these rates, casting an image of disorder and insecurity across entire regions.

63 Goldstein 1985. In addition, people who deal drugs are reluctant to commit violence, and violence can result from hyperviolent individuals or from "isolated episodes of disrespect" (Ayres and Ancrum 2023; Treadwell and Kelly 2023, 280; Rios 2011). To be sure, drug companies rely on police violence to protect private property, and corporate actors regularly engage in criminal conspiracy without being referred to as "gangs" (Treadwell and Kelly 2023).

64 Purnell 2021, 154–155.

65 Martin 2014. As a reminder from the introduction, the police and military have always blurred, given that they both extend the state's monopoly of violence to maintain capitalist order (Neocleous 2021).

66 Vitale 2017; M. Alexander 2012.

67 K. Williams 2023.

68 D. Gilmore 2009, 5.

69 Altheide 2003, 39.

70 Feldman 2004, 74. See Turner and Milburn (2024, 14–15) for paraphrasing.

71 Grégoire Chamayou (2012, 89) describes police as a "hunting institution," tasked with "tracking, arresting, and imprisoning." See Turner and Milburn 2024. Within a settler-colonial context, hunting is perceived as "adventure" and is constitutive of the killing of Indigenous people and the capture and enslavement of Africans (Dunbar-Ortiz 2018).

   Of further note, while popular coverage of the international drug trade can be informative in outlining trade routes, delivery styles, and surveillance techniques, it largely offers a drama of heroic interagency collaboration between federal, state, and local police who take down evil drug kingpins. This is evident, for instance, in reporting of the DEA's "stalking" (Feuer 2020) and "hunting" (Riley 2019) of the Sinaloa cartel leader Joaquin "El Chapo" Guzman as well as in the documentation of police tracking down the Xalisco boys of the Cártel de Jalisco Neuvo Generación, who delivered black-tar heroin "like pizza" across the Midwest (Quinones 2015).

72 Author's field notes, October 2017. As Ian Loader (1997, 3) reminds us, "popular attachment to policing is principally *affective* in character, something which people evince a deep emotional commitment to and which is closely integrated with their sense of self."

73 While drug seizure weights dropped from 2021 to 2023, the weight for fentanyl increased from 11,201 pounds in 2021 to 14,700 pounds in 2022 and to 27,023 pounds in 2023 (US CBP 2024). Similarly, the capture of Joaquin "El Chapo" Guzman did not stem the international drug trade. On January 31, 2019, the same day closing arguments were made in the trial of Guzman, "border officials made a startling announcement: They had just seized the largest load of fentanyl ever found in the United States" (Feuer 2020, 229). In *Drug Warrior*, the DEA special agent Jack Riley (2019, 50) also recognizes the futility of taking down large-scale drug kingpins, despite still espousing such enforcement practices. Riley notes that after the Colombian kingpin Pablo Escobar was killed in a police shootout on December 2, 1993, the Colombian Cali Cartel "leaped into the void," and with the waning of the Colombian drug cartel, the Sinaloa Cartel "stepped in to fill the void" (2019, 53, 68).

74 Borrelli 2020a. The task force made a 2018 drug seizure of $1 million worth of fentanyl, heroin, and meth. In the 2022 operation, police seized $27,000 worth of fentanyl.

75 Linnemann 2022, 193.

76 Garza 2020, 30.

CHAPTER 3. CARING COPS

1 PAARI, n.d.-a.

2 NYS Senate 2016.

3 PAARI, n.d.-b; LEAD, n.d.

4 Fatsis and Lamb 2022, 53; Foucault 1979.

5 Broome County, n.d.-a. (emphasis added).

6 Kaba and Ritchie 2022, 161; Fatsis and Lamb 2022; McQuade and Neocleous 2020.

7 Petersen 2024, 16; Mawby 2013.

8 PAARI 2015. The sheriff's PAARI program (PAARI 2016b) was called SARI (Sheriff Assisted Recovery Initiative). It reserved two beds at the Broome County Addiction Crisis Center (ACC) (Schwarz 2017).

9 Borrelli and Roby 2016.

10 PAARI 2016a.

11 Spencer 2009, 223.

12 Roby 2016a.

13 Staff 2016.

14 Borrelli 2015a.

15 Local reporting documented, "The rest of the funds would be distributed to local police for undercover operations and advanced computer equipment" (Borrelli 2018b).

16 As was confirmed in the local news, "Two of the witnesses who bought the heroin [leading to the arrests] have signed up for his Operation S.A.F.E. treatment program" (*Binghamton Homepage* 2016a).

17 It should be added that police's use of confidential informants can put people at risk of violent retaliation. As Derecka Purnell (2021, 142) reminds us, "Being a snitch is such a violation of street code that it could lead to the grave; hence the phrases 'snitches get stitches' and 'snitches get ditches.'" Nevertheless, police support for treatment has made more reasonable the use of confidential informants. Sam Quinones (2021, 211) documents Terry Sneary, the sheriff department's chief narcotics expert in Hardin County, Texas, as explaining the importance of supporting treatment for confidential informants: "We've started taking a closer look to see if we can offer [confidential informants] some help. . . . In the past, they were working with us, helping us take down a dealer, but then we were walking away. We knew we would encounter them again before long."

18 Mbembe 2019, 53.

19 A newspaper photo of Terrance "Money" Wise's arrest by two officers (discussed in chapter 2) provided a visual depiction of the police capture of a Black outsider dealer (Borrelli 2016g).

20 Linnemann 2017, 60.

21 Dunbar-Ortiz 2018, 127.

22 Roby 2016d.

23 Broome County 2017, 30.

24 Roby 2016d; see Borrelli 2016a.

25 *Binghamton Homepage* 2016b.

26 Roby 2016b.

27 Linnemann 2022, 69.

28 Mawby 2013.

29 Collins et al. 2015a, 2015b, 2017; Malm et al. 2020; Beckett 2022, 231; Clifasefi et al. 2016, 2017; Clifasefi and Collins 2016; Beckett 2014.

30 King 2019, 149.

31 Szalavitz 2016, 264.

32 Szalavitz 2016, 263.

33 Cornwell had a similar program to LEAD called Treatment Alternative to Prosecution. Those who were "charged with misdemeanor or lower charges such as petit larceny, or drug possession that are fueled by their substance abuse dependency" could avoid prosecution if they complete ninety days of treatment (Borrelli 2018a).

34 City of Ithaca 2016; Bright 2017.

35 Covert 2017 (parentheses in original in first excerpt).

36 LEAD 2017a. In 2020, the bureau updated the "Core Principles for Policing Role." The excerpts cited here remained in the document as of 2020, with the only difference being the deletion that it is not a "get out of jail free card" (LEAD 2020a).

37 LEAD 2017b. This text remained in the 2020 "Core Principles for Prosecutor Role" for the updated document (LEAD 2020b).

38 Beckett 2014, 31.

39 According to promotional material in Albany, New York (n.d.), the goals of LEAD are to:
    • Reorient government's response to safety, disorder and health-related problems.
    • Improve public safety and public health through research-based, health-oriented, and harm reduction interventions.
    • Reduce the number of people entering the criminal justice system for low-level offenses related to drug use, mental health, sex work, and extreme poverty.
    • Undo racial disparities at the front-end of the criminal justice system.
    • Sustain funding for alternative interventions by capturing and reinvesting criminal justice system savings.
    • Strengthen the relationship between law enforcement and the community.

40 DOJ 1994; Schenwar and Law 2020, 156.

41 Schenwar and Law 2020; Albany, New York, n.d.

42 Correia and Wall 2022, 189.

43 Correia and Wall 2022, 19.

44 Bell 1980.

45 Beckett 2008, 1.

46 Bluher 2018.

47 NYS DOH 2021.

48 Hamilton et al. 2021. The New York State 911 Good Samaritan law reads as follows: "A person who, in good faith, seeks health care for someone who is experiencing a drug or alcohol overdose or other life threatening medical emergency shall not be charged or prosecuted for a controlled substance offense under this article or a cannabis offense under article two hundred twenty-two of this title, other than an offense involving sale for consideration or other benefit or gain" (NYS Senate 2021).

49 Skelos 2011; Netherland 2023, 53–54.

50 McClellan et al. 2018; Lupick 2022, 187.

51 NYS DOH 2021.

52 R. Gilmore 2007, 28.

53 Netherland 2023, 89.

54 Stenersen et al. 2024.

55 Lupick 2022, 187. Interviewee Gabi, who worked at a local syringe-service program, mentioned that the restrictions made people nervous but viewed the law as an overall success: "It still makes people nervous to call 911, but it has been pretty successful in my experience. I know that a lot of our clients, if there's an overdose, will call 911. I'd say probably like, probably, half of everyone calls 911 in the case of an overdose of who I've talked to, which is pretty good. But it doesn't cover things like a warrant out for your arrest or parole violation or probation violation, so you know, it still prevents people from calling. But for the most part, it's good, but also with the policing thing."

56 Research shows that police generally hold negative views about people who use drugs (Kruis et al. 2022).

57 Kavanaugh 2022, 141.

58 Smiley-McDonald et al. 2022, 6. The police who were interviewed had mixed opinions, with some claiming that "angry or violent reactions" were "atypical" (Smiley-McDonald et al. 2022, 6).

59 Palmer 2020; Kavanaugh 2022, 45.

60 Smiley-McDonald et al. 2022, 6–7.

61 Kavanaugh 2022, 141.

62 Linnemann 2022.

63 Lupick 2022, 109–110, 168–169.

64 Author's field notes, February 2017.

65 Kavanaugh 2022, 144.

66 Seigel 2018, 10.

67 In *Ending Mass Incarceration*, Katherine Beckett (2022, 241) introduces LEAD 2.0, or JustCARE. JustCARE was established in 2020 when organizers cited issues with police presence in the original LEAD program; so they decided to operate *without them*. Access is not based on arrest or police recommendation, no drug testing is involved, and JustCARE focuses on reducing police contact, particularly for unsheltered people of color. The program utilizes community-based frameworks for participant outreach and offers "permanent housing and support services." Participants "choose for themselves whether, when, and how much to share about their drug use with their case manager or outreach responder." As Beckett (2022, 244) reports of the program, "During JustCARE's first wave of operations, nearly three-fourths—73.5 percent—of the people offered housing and support from a JustCARE provider were people of color."

CHAPTER 4. CARING COURTS

1 Borrelli 2017d.

2 Borrelli 2018c.

3 The judge's statements perhaps reflect a kind of "feminized blamelessness," in which white women who use or deal drugs are viewed as deserving "gentleness and compassion," as in need of "protection *by* and *from* the state" (Daniels et al. 2018, 339).

4 Kaba 2017.

5 Broome County, n.d.-b.

6 By the end of 2021, nearly 3.7 million people, or one in sixty-nine adults, were on probation or parole in the US (Pew Charitable Trust 2023; BJS 2009). In 2021, 30 percent of adults were on parole and 26 percent were on probation for a drug-related offense (Kaeble 2023).

7 Wexler and Winick 1996. Drug courts have their origin in 1960s problem-solving courts, which utilized courts for mental health, juvenile delinquency, and domestic violence (Tiger 2011).

8 Quinones 2021, 201. Quinones (2021, 355) tells of two participants, Melissa Carter and Jesse Clevenger, "who stopped using when they were forced into drug court." "I wouldn't have got clean," Clevenger said, "if I didn't have that ultimatum."

9 White House 2011, 2022a, n.d.; Sacco 2018; DHHS 2024.

10 National Treatment Court Resource Center 2024.

11 NYS UCS, n.d.-a; Punch et al. 2022. New York State's first drug court was established in Rochester in 1995 by Chief Judge Judith Kaye. She argued that courts were not "making a dent" in drug crime. Within five years, twenty courts were in full operation (Feinblatt et al. 2000, 278). Drug courts have also served political commitments to roll back the 1973 Rockefeller drug laws (Mancuso 2010).

12 NYS UCS, n.d.-d.

13 Broome County 2017, 30. As with police-based treatment, the drug court has restricted access for sex offenders and for "accused drug dealers or violent criminal defendants" (Borrelli 2016e).

14 Moore 2011, 259.

15 Given policy restrictions against computers and audio recording, I wrote down my observations in a notebook, quoting and paraphrasing to the best of my ability (Revier 2021a, 921).

16 Moore 2011, 257; Foucault 2007, 172.

17 Moore 2011, 259.

18 Nolan 2001, 85.

19 Moore 2011, 257.

20 D. Moore et al. 2011. Such regulation is based on the Pavlovian idea that "an external cue, such as a certain location, sounds, or other sensory experiences, becomes associated with a behavior" (Belenko and Spohn 2014, 52; Belenko et al. 2011).

21 Kilgore 2022, 47. Of note, e-bracelets can have technological malfunctions, and users pay service fees and fines (Cowles 2019, 232).

22 Kilgore 2022, 24.

23 Szalavitz 2016, 181.

24 Samaritan Daytop Village, n.d.

25 Fletcher 2013. This was especially pronounced in Synanon, the first addiction-focused therapeutic community, which was opened in 1958 by an AA member, Charles Dederich Sr. It employed attack therapy, silence, shunning, and sleep and food deprivation and was rife with physical and mental abuse. See Szalavitz 2016; Kaye 2019.

26 Schenwar and Law 2020, 18; see also Kaba and Ritchie 2022, 156. Kerwin Kaye (2019, 225) observed in a New York City inpatient treatment center, as summarized well by Carl Fisher (2022, 224), "Staff regularly berated clients, humiliated people in front of groups, and called them names like 'dope fiends.' In the worst example, after one disciplinary infraction, the staff ransacked all the residents' rooms, overturning mattresses and dumping out their possessions, then made them clean it all up—according to the facility's usual militaristic, spotless standard—until well after midnight."

27 Campbell 2004, 78. The Binghamton drug court judge asserted to participants that drug testing "is right in the heart and integrity of the program," stating, "You need to keep clean, and one way is to test."

28 Schenwar and Law 2020, 100.

29 Twelve-step programs are not necessarily appealing for many people (see Lupick 2022, 43–44). Mandating twelve-step attendance also violates the First Amendment's Establishment Clause, which "prohibits governmental bodies from preferring religion over non-religion or vice versa" (Cowles 2019, 45). Nevertheless, twelve-step meetings are often the only ones available in many communities.

30 Russell et al. 2022, 152.

31 NYS UCS, n.d.-a.

32 Narrative habitus, as Jennifer Fleetwood (2016, 181) defines it, is "the internalisation of the narrative doxa pertaining to the field, including vocabulary, narrative formats, tropes, discursive formats and subject positions etc." See also Presser 2016. On shifting penal subjectivity, see Donohue and Moore 2009.

33 Carr 2010, 15.

34 Carr 2010, 2.

35 Nolan 2001.

36 Moore 2007.

37 NYS UCS, n.d.-c (emphasis added). In addition, New York State recognizes drug court as being offered to "defendants facing felony or misdemeanor charges where *drug addiction* is a component of their offense." NYS UCS, n.d.-a (emphasis added).

38 Keane 2002, 69.

39 Burns and Peyrot 2003.

40 NYS UCS, n.d.-c.

41 The judge's forecasting echoes cautionary temperance tales of the "drunkard" progressing "to the poorhouse and grave" (Room 2003, 229).

42 Tiger 2013; Gowan and Whetstone 2012, 80.

43 McKim 2017, 75.

44 Revier 2021a.

45 A. Frank 2010.

46 NYS UCS, n.d.-c.

47 Gowan and Whetstone 2012, 81.

48 Nolan 2001, 73.

49 Murphy 2015.

50 Kaye 2019, 217.

51 Burns and Peyrot 2003. After all, addiction is largely considered a disease of *denial* (Carr 2010, 11).

52 D. Anderson 2015.

53 Ugelvik 2014.

54 DPA 2011. Whites are also more likely to be accepted into and graduate from drug court (Nicosia et al. 2013; McKean and Warren-Gordon 2011) and are disproportionately sent to less restrictive outpatient care (Kaye 2019). Furthermore, cities that have established drug courts have experienced increased misdemeanor drug arrests per year (Lilley 2017; Lilly et al. 2020), and cities with larger populations of color "were more likely to create drug courts, but once established, drug courts were associated with a higher arrest rate for Black—but not White—residents" (Beckett 2022, 131; Lilley et al. 2019). One study found that a quarter of women participants in a St. Louis, Missouri, drug court experienced sexual misconduct by police (Cottler et al. 2014).

55 NYS UCS, n.d.-d.

56 Kaye 2019. Sam Quinones (2021, 215) identifies participants as "raw material" for employers: "American businesses could extract competitive advantage, help their bottom line and their towns by hiring recovering addicts—this new raw material, rejected by others."

57 E. Summerson Carr (2010, 3) documents treatment clients as "flipping the script"; this occurs when participants "formally replicat[e] prescribed ways of speaking about themselves and their problems without investing in the *content* of those scripts."

58 Kaye 2019, 142.

59 Kaye 2019, 24; Hartman 2022.

60 W. Brown 1995, 23; see also Turner and Milburn 2024, 6.

61 NYS UCS, n.d.-a.

62 Tiger 2013, paraphrased by Beckett 2022, 133.

63 Eighty-five percent of parolees in New York wind up incarcerated for technical violations (Columbia University Justice Lab 2020; Blakinger 2022, 265; Council of State Governments Justice Center 2019).

64 Michelle spoke of the house visit in full: "[They came in] like screaming. I'm like, 'okay,' you know? 'I'm not the one that's in trouble. Keep it down.' But—and they just come in your house, and they look around. But, I mean, if he's not doing anything wrong, I have nothing to hide. . . . I mean, she was like also disrespectful. She's like, 'What are you chewing in your mouth? Spit it out.' And I'm thinking, 'You're in my house,' you know? 'I'm not the one that did anything wrong.'"

Lucas's sister, Alex, added that her brother was unable to leave the county, which she felt impeded his recovery. "My brother has wanted to leave Broome County, but they don't—they won't let him. This is obviously a very toxic—this has been going on for like, I don't know, eight years, nine years now, and he can't leave. He can't start over. It doesn't matter how many rehabs he goes to. Every person he knows—you could walk down the street, and like ten—he knows every other person." In this sense, probation works *against* drug courts' spatial regulation, with regard to prioritizing participants not going to places that trigger drug use (D. Moore et al. 2011).

65 Drug courts have been shown to reduce recidivism from 50 to 38 percent (Mitchell et al. 2012). Of note, a focus on recidivism reinforces a criminal-addict identity by linking together drug use, crime, addiction, and recovery. Indeed, when defining recidivism, the National Institute of Justice (NIJ, n.d.) uses the phrase "*relapse* into criminal behavior," further entangling discourses of addiction and crime (emphasis added). The discursive fusing of crime and addiction is also evident in the city drug court's mission of "enhancing public *safety*" (NYS UCS, n.d.-b; emphasis added).

66 Gill et al. 2018. Indeed, the incarceration rate in Broome County decreased in 2020 due to releases from COVID-19 restrictions and the 2019 bail reform, which eliminated cash bail for most misdemeanors and nonviolent felonies. A month after bail reform went into effect, in February 2020, the average daily jail population fell by 25 percent, from 427 to 322 (Vera Institute of Justice 2021). Nevertheless, with these changes, one could still be sentenced for drug-related charges and be sent to jail on probation *and* drug court violations. In an analysis of pretrial detention outside of New York City, Jaeok Kim et al. (2021, 21) speculate that "almost 60 percent of pretrial admissions were for either misdemeanor or nonviolent felony charges after bail reform."

67 Martin 2019a. See also the case of Thomas Husar, who died in the jail after being incarcerated for a probation violation (Borrelli 2020b).

68 Author's field notes, February 2019; Norton 2019.

CHAPTER 5. CARING CAGES

1 Author's field notes, September 2017.

2 The Broome County expansion follows trends in jail growth across upstate New York (Pragacz 2016; Norton 2018; Subramanian et al. 2018).

3   Broome County 2025.

4   Broome County, n.d.-a.

5   Vera Institute of Justice 2019, 2023. In 2015, Broome County incarcerated 467 per 100,000 residents, which was 120 percent higher than New York City (at 357 per 100,000; Henrichson et al. 2018). Even with a drop in the incarceration rate in 2020, Broome County maintained a rate of 273 per 100,000, which was over twice the state average (at 101 per 100,000; Vera Institute of Justice 2021).

6   Roby 2015.

7   *Binghamton Homepage* 2018.

8   In 2018, the New York State Senate's Heroin Task Force approved $4 million for addiction services across New York jails, with $400,000 earmarked for Broome County (Spectrum News Staff 2018). In 2021, Governor Kathy Hochul passed legislation that mandates medication-assisted opioid treatment (MOAD) access in the state's forty-four prisons and sixty-two jails (NYS 2021). Of note, the New York State Sheriffs' Association opposed the legislation, saying in a memo that the "decision whether to offer [medication-assisted treatment] is one that resides, and should remain with, the Sheriff" (Norris 2023d). Thus, carceral humanism operates through a variety of competing interests (Kilgore 2014). As Justin Helepololei (2024, 288) explains of what he refers to as the "progressive jail assemblage," it is "a far less coherent, often conflicting convergence of actors, institutions, and policies."

9   Broome County, n.d.-a.

10 Irwin (1985) 2013, 2.

11 New York Heritage, n.d.; French, n.d.

12 Norton et al. 2024b, 14; Miller 2014.

13 Martin 2022a.

14 Davis 2003; Price 2015a.

15 Kilgore 2014; Schept 2015.

16 Walter (2019) contrasts jail health care with the World Health Organization's (WHO's) definition of health as "a state of complete physical, mental, and social wellbeing, and not merely the absence of disease or infirmity" (WHO 2022).

17 Whites made up 82 percent of the county population in 2023 but made up 60 percent of the jail population (Vera Institute of Justice 2023; Martin 2018). Of note, 98 percent of the Binghamton Police Department (BPD) in 2016 were white (Borrelli 2016b).

18 As Frantz Fanon (1967, 168) states of the usefulness of Blackness to explain white deviance, "If I behave like a man with morals, I am not black. Hence the saying in Martinique that a wicked white man has the soul of a n****r."

19 Macy 2018, 117–118.

20 Macy 2012b.

21 Keane 2002, 69.

22 Eyre 2016.

23 J. Eaton 2017.

24 Quinones 2017.

25 Quinones 2017.

26 Quinones 2021, 272–273.

27 Quinones 2021, 252.

28 Macy 2022, 172.

29 National Sheriffs' Association and National Commission on Correctional Health Care 2018.

30 The letter was coordinated by the advocacy groups Fair and Just Prosecution and Law Enforcement Action Partnership (LEAP) (Filter Staff 2019; brackets in original). Indeed, in Hampden County, Massachusetts, Sheriff Nicholas Cocchi has utilized the state's involuntary civil commitment ordinances to incarcerate people "solely based on addiction" (Helepololei 2024, 291).

31 R. Gilmore 2022, 474.

32 K. Moore et al. 2019. Jail and prison treatment has been shown to decrease overdose death upon release, reduce disciplinary issues, and lessen rates of HIV and hepatitis C (Degenhardt et al. 2014; Lazarus et al. 2018; Stöver and Hariga 2016; Michaud and van der Meulen 2023).

33 It is important to consider how Megan's socioeconomic status contributed to her jail experience and subsequent recovery.

34 Macy 2022, 172–174.

35 Price 2015a, 17; Santos 2007, 48. Erving Goffman (1961, xiii) defines total institutions as being "cut off from the wider society for an appreciable period of time." Those who are incarcerated are *cut off* in a number of ways, although it should be noted that carceral spaces are never totally isolated entities (Gill et al. 2018). In the Broome County jail, there is no weekend visitation. Visitors must travel long hours and are restricted to a few hours a week, and visitation is often disrupted by lockdowns. The visitor must wait, be searched before entering, and be watched by correctional officers during the visit, making the visiting process itself a punishing experience. Interviewee Ray described visiting a woman he had been advocating for: "I made three visits to Steuben County. Three or four—I don't remember how many. But it's a long ride. It's a six-hour day. Essentially, an hour and a half out, and you have to get there an hour early. Because if you did not get there an hour early, you didn't get to see them. And you literally had to stand in line, get in line, and stand for an hour. . . . So, I get there early enough, stand in line. And then you get a one-hour visit, [a] noncontact visit." Additionally, phone tablet communication is costly, and the Broome County jail eliminated in-person visitation for two years after initial COVID-19 protocols (JUST 2022). As a final note, jails can also limit and restrict research with those who are incarcerated (see Price 2015a).

36 M. Brown 2009. There are several ways the experiences of incarcerated people are suppressed. While the New York Inmate Grievance Program mandates a grievance officer every twenty-four hours, the complainant must "attempt to get the issue resolved with the housing officer" (Broome County Office of the Sheriff 2013, 2023). Grievance officers are often not present, and incarcerated people seeking

forms are at times penalized by correctional officers (Martin 2024). Interviewee Ron spoke of such retaliation: "Good luck getting a grievance through. They're all buddies. . . . If you grieve one officer, you're gonna end up in the box [solitary confinement]." In addition, 99 percent of grievances were denied from 2017 to 2022 by the New York State Commission of Corrections (Martin 2022b; NYS Comptroller 2017).

Correctional officers also influence the ability of incarcerated people to bear witness to state violence. Ron stated when referring to correctional officers beating the incarcerated Salladin Barton, whose case I review in this chapter, "When the sheriffs come into the pod, like more than one of them for an incident like that, you have to get off your gate, you know, or they're gonna give you another thirty days in solitary confinement. If you're caught . . . looking out your cell watching them, they're gonna give you another thirty days in the box. . . . So you have to lay down on your bed and stare at the ceiling . . . because they don't want anybody to see what's really going on. They don't want anyone to see the truth." In this regard, state officials organize a visual field, where they make it difficult for state institutions and actors to be seen by researchers, advocates, family, community members, and those who are in conflict with the law (Schept 2014).

37 Broome County Office of the Sheriff 2013, 2023.
38 Roby 2016c.
39 Price 2015b.
40 *Taejon Vega v. Broome County, Richard Hrebin, Corey Fowler, and Daniel Weir,* Case No. 9:21-cv-788 (N.D.N.Y. July 10, 2021).
41 Russell et al. 2022, 153; Price 2017. See Chris Gelardi (2022) on "therapeutic" isolation in the wake of New York's Humane Alternatives to Long-Term Solitary Confinement (HALT) Act, which went into effect in 2022.
42 From collecting jail letters and visiting incarcerated people, advocates cited the private medical provider as restricting inhalers, seizure medication, blood pressure medication, heart medication, hearing aids, glasses, insulin, hormones, and antianxiety and antidepression medication. In 2011, for instance, Alvin Rios was not properly detoxed off alcohol and benzodiazepines. A correctional officer found him in a cell "face down and shaking." He died of "cardiac arrhythmia produced by cardiomyopathy," an abnormal heart rhythm stemming from the deterioration of the heart muscle. The county settled with his family for $62,000 (Reilly 2014).
43 Johnson 2001. Imani explained of the intake process in full,
Essentially the second you walk in, you go into intake. They sit you down, and they fill out a bunch of paperwork, asking you a bunch of questions, looking for tattoos. Obviously, they pat you down and get all of your possessions out of your pockets and stuff. . . . Once you're done doing that, they'll put you in the clinical bullpen, which is this extra-big cell . . . which has some benches-type thing and a couple toilets. They'll take you back out of

that when they're ready to get your fingerprints and mug shot. Then they stick you back in there.

Then you'll go talk to the intake nurse, who'll ask you about any diseases that you have, prescriptions, all of that type of stuff, put you back in the bullpen until you get your jumpsuit. And you get the one that you put on. You get an extra one. You get two shirts, one of those that go on, two pairs of socks, one of them that goes on, two pairs of underwear, one of 'em that goes on. So you basically have one full change of clothes and then everything else you're wearing. And then they'll give you a sheet, two blankets, and . . . the "bed roll," quote/unquote.

44 Feeley 1979; Armstrong 2018; Eife and Kirk 2021.
45 Irwin (1985) 2013, 68–69; Goffman 1961. Keri Blakinger (2022, 194) writes of her fight for basic hygiene with women she was incarcerated with: "The most valuable commodity here was toilet paper—and since we only got five rolls a month, we collected magazines and newspapers to use as backup, like magpies conniving our way into basic hygiene."
46 Arnold and Pleus 2018.
47 Broome County Office of the Sheriff 2013, 2023.
48 In 2018, approximately 42 percent of inmate sexual victimization in adult correctional facilities were committed by staff (Buehler 2021).
49 Davis 2003, 83. The Supreme Court determined that pretrial detention is not punishment and strip searches are permitted for safety and security measures. They are therefore considered not to violate the Fourteenth Amendment's Due Process Clause (*Bell v. Wolfish*, 441 U.S. 520 [1979]).

To be sure, visitors are also subjected to humiliating searches. John Edgar Wideman's ([1984] 2020, 210) writing on a prison in Pittsburgh, Pennsylvania, is revealing:

After the solid steel door, before the barred, locked gate into the visiting area proper, each visitor must pass through a metal-detecting machine. The reason for such a security measure is clear; the extreme sensitivity of the machine is less easily explained. Unless the point is inflicting humiliation on visitors. Especially women visitors whose underclothes contain metal stays and braces, women who wear intimate jewelry they never remove from their bodies. Grandmothers whose wedding rings are imbedded in the flesh of their fingers. When the machine bleeps, everything it discovers must go. You say it's a wire in your bra, lady. Well, I'm sorry about that but you gotta take it off. Of course the women have a choice. They can strip off the offending garment or ornament, and don one of the dowdy smocks the state provides for such contingencies. Or they can go back home.

50 Blakinger 2022, 248. The facility has also provided degraded clothing. As Bill Martin (2019b) reported, "Persons working in laundry confirm that underwear is old, stained by body fluids, and not adequately cleaned. Bras, laundry workers have stated, are so old, torn, and dirty that they are almost unrecognizable as they

go through the wash." On top of this, in 2019 the jail removed "the ability to buy from the commissary clean underwear, bras, and thermal shirts."

51 NYCLU 2022. In 2023, Holland settled with Broome County for $160,000. The county has since committed to a series of gender-affirming policies, including access to medical care free from discrimination and assigning transgender people to units on the basis of their gender identity (NYCLU 2023). While certainly a victory, such policies do suit carceral humanist tendences toward gender-responsive care, and here transgender-responsive care, which does not address the circumstances in which gender-nonconforming people are policed and incarcerated in the first place (Kilgore 2014). Indeed, transgender people of color face particularly high rates of carceral abuse (SRLP et al. 2021; Oberholtzer 2017).

52 Ross 1998, 128.

53 Kaba 2018, 190. Kaba develops Connie Chung's (2011) concept of (un)mothering.

54 Roberts 2022. Indeed, Indigenous children constitute less than 1 percent of children in the US but constitute roughly 25 to 50 percent of children removed from families (Potawatomi Nation 2021). Black children comprise nearly 25 percent of kids in foster care despite constituting approximately 13 percent of children in the US (Purnell 2021, 269–270).

55 Price 2015a, 23; V. Law 2015; O. Patterson (1982) 2018.

56 Price 2015a; Walter 2019, 18.

57 Davis 2003; Hartman 2022, 148. The enslaved person was deemed by the courts to serve not just for economic profit but for "the *joy* of the master in the sexual conquest of the slave." Higginbotham 1989, 694 (emphasis added); Hartman 2022, 149.

58 hooks 2012; Davis 2003; Ross 2004; Díaz-Cotto 2006.

59 Purnell 2021, 54; hooks 2004. Hartman (2022, 139), too, makes note of how "the castration and assault of slave men" was encompassed in the range of sexual violence that overseers imposed.

60 Binswanger et al. 2007; Merrall et al. 2010; Lim et al. 2012; Ranapurwala et al. 2018; Degenhardt et al. 2014.

61 Mars et al. 2014.

62 As Katherine Beckett (2022, 224) points out, "Jail often makes matters worse by disrupting benefits, medication, employment, and housing, families, and by creating the mark of a criminal conviction and exposing people to additional trauma. Even short jail stays decrease employment and tax-related government benefits, increase homelessness, and exacerbate racial inequities."

63 NYS, n.d.-a.

64 Lubben 2023.

65 Price 2016.

66 Price 2016, 89; NYS OTDA 2011.

67 McQuade and Neocleous 2020; Soss et al. 2011. John Halushka (2020, 233) describes formerly incarcerated interviewees as having to manage "overlapping entanglements across a fragmented network of bureaucracy." As he elaborates, "Formerly-incarcerated men must repeatedly engage with parole, public assis-

tance agencies, transitional housing facilities, and community-based service providers to maintain freedom and access food, shelter, and rehabilitative services."

68 Norris 2023a.

69 The New York State reentry program ABLE (Advocacy, Betterment, Learning, Empowerment), which runs out of DSS, "specialize[s] in employment, and immediate needs stabilization" (ABLE 2025).

70 Miller 2021, 228. Interviewee Mary spoke of these approaches in Broome County reentry programming: "They don't call it 'behavioral modification.' They don't call it 'CBT.' They don't call it 'cognitive behavioral therapy.' They call it 'thinking for change.' It's that introspective work, which is very hard to do, and I guess, I mean, if they think of one behavior that they could change and make things different, I guess maybe it'll be successful. But to me, it just seems imposing on people."

I have made a similar observation regarding evidence-based cognitive behavioral therapy (CBT) programming in US prisons. Such programs do not focus on structural conditions that relate to drug use, crime, and incarceration but on participants' "criminal thinking errors" and "criminal lifestyle." I refer to the use of CBT within carceral settings as "carceral CBT" (Revier 2023; see also Fox 1999).

71 Miller 2021, 234; Soss et al. 2011, 241.

72 Purser 2021.

73 Price 2016, 85. The "ultimate goal" of ABLE "is of reducing recidivism, rebuilding lives and communities, and enhancing public safety" (NYS, n.d.-b). On receiving jail funding from New York State, Senator Fred Akshar also stressed the dual goals of *recidivism* and *productivity*: "Study after study shows that these services substantially reduce recidivism and more effectively help individuals who find themselves incarcerated get back on the right track. By receiving treatment while on the inside, they're put in a vastly better position to stay in recovery and become more productive members of society on the outside" (NYS Senate 2018).

74 Miller and Stuart 2017, 532. Carceral citizenship echoes the condition of emancipated African Americans. Hartman describes freed Black people as having burdened citizenship, as they "occupied the precarious position of being free but without the basic rights of citizenship" (2022, 307–308). Such burdened citizenship facilitated coerced labor, judicial and extrajudicial violence, and an emphasis on moral cultivation severed from property and civil rights.

75 Interviewee Jim argued that, while the jail had offered a shot of Naltrexone (brand name Vivitrol) to suppress cravings upon his release, a lack of treatment services merely prolonged the chance of a fatal overdose: "They're talking about [how] they're gonna shoot people with Vivitrol before they leave jail. Great idea, but unless you got them set up in an outpatient, too, you're fucking them, because that means they're just gonna get thirty extra days clean from when they leave jail. . . . So they're basically getting [an] extra thirty days of life"; Author's field notes, 2019.

76 See Judah Schept (2015, 10) on carceral habitus as "the corporal and discursive inscription of penal logics into individual and community bodies."

77 Quinones 2017.

78 See also Irwin (1985) 2013; Price 2015a; Jeffreys 2018; Venters 2019; Friday 2022; Klein and Klein 2022. I documented an instance of ordinary violence the first time I visited an incarcerated person with a fellow advocate. I was in the jail's parking lot debriefing with him. We saw the jail's physician, who committed numerous abuses, walking to his vehicle. I debriefed in my field notes:

> It is bright and warm outside: And I feel hatred toward him. I think of institutional harms: oppressive forces, weaved through structures and histories of violence. But here is the doctor—*the doctor* I've heard so much about—walking to his vehicle. The moment captures a sense of freedom contrasted with the confinement of those incarcerated. The vehicle he will leave with is funded by the pain he has caused for so many. His gait—his ability to move across institutional divides—feels like a flaunting of state power: it is not the abusive police officer on the street, captured on camera, but a doctor walking to his vehicle in a parking lot. I feel helpless. (Author's field notes, May 2018)

79 Helepololei 2024; Ugelvik 2014, 52.

80 For review, see Miller 2021, 196–197; see also E. Patterson 2013.

81 Bennett 2008; Berger et al. 2017.

82 Litigants have relied on the Eighth Amendment's protection against cruel and unusual punishment, the Fourteenth Amendment's Equal Protection Clause, and the Americans with Disabilities Act (see Arnold 2019; Marton and de la Guéronnière 2019; Jackson 2019; ACLU 2019). See also Blum 2024.

83 *Robinson v. California*, 370 U.S. 660 (1962). In *Powell v. Texas*, 392 U.S. 514 (1968), the Supreme Court concluded that individuals like "chronic alcoholics" are still subject to laws such as those against public intoxication.

84 APA 2013; PPI 2024.

85 McLellan et al. 2000.

86 SAMHSA 2024. About 40 percent of people with a mental health issue (NIDA 2018) and 20 percent of people with a mental illness (SAMHSA 2011) have been identified as having a substance use disorder; 61 percent of people with bipolar I and 48 percent of people with bipolar II will meet the criteria for SUD during their lifetime (Vornik and Brown 2006; Lupick 2022, 9).

87 Lewis 2021, 22. Of note, one in every four people killed by police has a mental illness (Fuller et al. 2015; see Vitale 2017, 77). Policing, in addition, *is disabling*, as police produce trauma and injury during, for instance, drug raids and protest suppression (Purnell 2021, 218–220).

88 Norris 2013b. Of note, while the New York 2021 legislation mandated peer support in jails, Spencer Norris (2023c) found a lack of "guidelines for what they should look like," and there were no "legal protections against discrimination for peers based on their criminal record." See also Helepololei 2024; and Michaud and van der Meulen 2023.

89 Giblin 2023.

90 By 2010, Suboxone sales reached over $1 billion (*CESAR Fax* 2012), with a recent loss of revenue due to the release of generic products (Stanton 2015). More

broadly, as Helena Hansen and colleagues (2023a, 23) note, "Pharmaceutical, biotechnology, and health care industries together make up the largest sector of the US economy."

91 Gilmore and Gilmore 2008, 142.

92 Hartman 2022, 6. Neocleous (2021, 208–209) applies the term "legal fetishism" to refer to the notion that "law" is "a background assumption, operating as an ambiguous standard from which the police, as 'law enforcers,' are assumed to deviate." Legal fetishism presumes that police follow an abstract tapestry of law rather than law acting as another tool for *policing order*. As Neocleous (2021, 212) concludes, "Police practices are designed to conform to and prioritize order, not law, as the judiciary and police have long known."

93 Mattlin 2022, xx; W. Eaton 1990.

94 Kaba and Hayes 2018.

95 Ferrell 2013, 258.

CONCLUSION

1 Author's field notes, 2019.

2 Szalavitz 2016, 263.

3 Christie 2007, 21.

4 Szalavitz 2016, 264–265.

5 Szalavitz 2016, 263.

6 Macy 2022.

7 Schenwar and Law 2020, 17.

8 Rebecca Tiger (2013, 8) reminds us in her critical drug court research that reform has been "foundational to the development of the modern penal system." See also Rothman 2017.

9 Kaba 2020; Vitale 2017, 27.

10 Hayes and Kaba 2023, 247.

11 Thier 2020, 139. Even when legalized, the commodification of drugs sucks up the "free gifts" of nature through exploited labor—from coffee cultivation in South and Central America and barley growth for beer in North America to opium poppy picking in South Asia (Harvey 2017).

12 Berger et al. 2017. See Critical Resistance 2021.

13 Herzing 2015.

14 Kaba 2014.

15 Berger et al. 2017; Beckett 2022; Norton et al. 2024b.

16 See R. Gilmore 2015; Gottschalk 2014; Forman 2012; Beckett 2022.

17 Hampton 2024, 271. Hampton (2024, 272) furthermore adds that police "still have a crucial role in helping people access social support and health care," a point I have been critical of throughout this book.

18 Cowles 2019, 185.

19 Mbembe 2019, 38. Police, for instance, do not make people safer from sexual violence. Rape kits often sit on shelves, and police make an arrest for only 33 percent

of reported rapes, with the conviction and imprisonment rate being even lower (Purnell 2021, 175). Policing simply does not get at the roots of sexual violence within patriarchal capitalism.

20 Kaba and Hayes 2018. As I account for in the appendix, protesters at a rally at the Purdue Pharmaceutical headquarters yelled, "Lock them up!"

21 Hayes and Kaba 2023, 247.

22 Fatsis and Lamb 2022, 91.

23 Gilmore and Kilgore 2019.

24 See Brown and Schept 2017, 446; Hayes and Kaba 2023, 62; Vitale 2017. Without broader social investment, progressive drug policies do not adequately address drug-related violence. Consider the decriminalization of drugs. Decriminalization is defined as the removal or reduction of the criminal classification or status of a drug. The drug remains illegal, although "the legal system would not prosecute the person for the act," and "the penalties would range from no penalties at all to a civil fine" (LII 2022). Decriminalization has shown success in reducing overdoses in Portugal (Hart 2013). Nevertheless, without investment in public infrastructure, as Katherine Beckett (2022, 217–218) contends, decriminalization leaves the untested potency of drugs intact as well as the "unregulated competition among traffickers and dealers, all of which contributes to systemic, drug-related violence."

25 Hayes and Kaba 2023, 249. Consider the Drug User Liberation Front, or "DULF" for short. DULF was established between August 2022 and October 2023 in Vancouver, British Columbia. Organizers provide supervised consumption services and "rigorously tested cocaine, heroin, and methamphetamine at cost to club members" (Nyx and Kalicum 2024, 1). Since they are not exempt from Canada's Controlled Drugs and Substance Act, they have faced police scrutiny and were raided on October 25, 2023. Protesters showed up in the Downtown Eastside of Vancouver, British Columbia, on November 3, chanting, "Safe supply—or we die!"; "1-2-3—fuck the VPD!"; and "DULF saves lives!" (Godfrey 2023, 2024).

26 McHarris 2024. See also the interview with Lexi Peterson-Burge on nonpolice crisis intervention to offset carceral responses to Hurricane Katrina (Norton et al. 2024a, 139).

27 Hayes and Kaba 2023, 60. See also Schept 2022, 15; Hall et al. 1978.

28 Hay et al. 2013, 14.

29 Woodland 2023b, 81. Healing justice operates through three basic principles: Collective trauma is transformed collectively; there is no single model of care; and healing strategies are rooted in place and ancestral technologies (Page and Woodland 2023, 265). It should be noted that healing justice activists do not totally reject Western medicine, and many proponents work in the health-care industry. Rather, healing justice opposes the medical industrial complex (MIC), which operates to "surveil, police, and erase those seen as expendable, incurable, unfit, abnormal, or dangerous, as based on ableist and racist eugenic science" (Page and Woodland 2023, 265). As such, healing justice seeks to integrate elements of

Western medicine within community that honors culture and language and seeks
to address generational trauma linked to slavery, colonialism, and racial capitalism more broadly.

30 Gumbs 2023.

31 Purnell 2021, 210.

32 Purnell 2021, 107. As Robin D. G. Kelley (2002, 17) further explains, "These settle-
ments often existed on the run, in the hills or swamps just outside the plantation
economy. Africans tended to dominate these communities, and many sought to
preserve the cultures of their original homelands while combining different Old
and New World traditions. Over time, Africans adopted elements of various Native American cultures, and vice versa, and Europeans relied on aspects of these
cultures for their own survival."

33 McHarris 2024.

34 Purnell 2021, 143.

35 Harriet Tubman Collective 2017; Purnell 2021, 213. As Talila Lewis (2021, 42)
reminds us, "Abolition depends on racial, economic, and healing justice—all of
which depend on disability justice." See also Tastrom 2024.

36 See Lupick 2022, 236. Syringe-service programs have refrained from hiring people
who use drugs and have maintained restricted office hours (see Lupick 2022;
Vakharia 2024). The focus on risky use in dominant harm-reduction practices
also presumes the irrationality of people who use drugs. After all, as Carl Hart
(2021, 61) points out, "only a feebleminded soul would engage in an activity that
always produces harmful outcomes, as the term implies."

37 S. Hassan 2023, 86–87.

38 S. Hassan 2023, 87–88.

39 Raffo 2023, 159–160.

40 S. Hassan 2023, 88. As the nonbinary activist Prosperino puts it well, "We won't
have real harm reduction unless we defund the police" (Macy 2022, 131).

41 Woodland 2023a, 174.

42 In *Filter*, Louise Vincent (2018) rejects drug-induced-homicide laws when writing, "The outcome in drug-induced-homicide cases is two lives lost instead of
one—and a false appearance of retribution, justice, and revenge."

43 Milstein 2017, 4. See also Hayes and Kaba 2023, 152.

44 Garza 2020, 9.

45 Garza 2020; Butler 2004; Fraser et al. 2018.

46 Garza 2020, 7. Recognizing grief is paramount to work against the "habituation
to loss" within racial capitalism (Mbembe 2019, 38). As Hayes and Kaba (2023,
152) state, "If the public at large accepts preventable mass deaths as inevitable,
the system will maintain itself." In fact, as they continue, "Our oppressors
rely on our hesitation to feel for one another. They rely on our suppression of
empathy and grief and on the desensitization that often takes hold as a defense
mechanism in the face of so much suffering. They are hoping that the battery
of catastrophe we witness in real time will shorten our attention spans until

the fallen are forgotten in the blink of an eye." In regard to the overdose crisis, Ryan Hampton (2024, 7) adds sharply, "I do not accept the widespread deaths as endemic to our culture."

47 Kushner 2019.

48 Schenwar and Law 2020, 198.

49 Ewing 2019.

50 Matsuda 1989, 8. See D. Greene 1989.

51 See Purnell 2021, 82.

52 Arani 2022, 13.

53 As Hayes and Kaba (2023, 59) declare, "As organizers we must learn to conjure that social electricity even in relatively 'normal' times." After all, relatively "normal" times are rife with white supremacy's "quotidian routine of violence" (Hartman 2022, 66). And, as Purnell (2021, 264) adds, "As long as there have been people willing to destroy humans for a profit, there have been people resisting," with "spectacular and quotidian claims to live a healthy life."

54 Sarai 2024. In Mary O'Donovan's (2014, 296) Broome County fieldwork, she adopts David Harvey's (2012) work on the local and authentic to open space for oppositional movement building.

55 Martin 2020.

56 Samson 2017; Guest Contributor 2017.

57 Kilgore 2014.

58 Pragacz and Revier 2024, 80–81.

59 Pleus and Revier 2018; B. Smith 2018.

60 The harm-reduction specialist Gabi similarly asserted in our interview that a person should have the autonomy to make choices regarding use and have resources available to do so, whether they seek treatment or not. As she put it, "Addiction is an illness, and even if it's not, people should have the autonomy to make their own decisions and not have to die because of them."

61 Johnston 2018.

62 Sprout Distro 2017. Author's field notes, September 2018. Indeed, police have not made me, even as a white male, feel particularly safe, not just as a protestor but as a victim. When walking home with a friend after a night of heavy drinking and MDMA use, we were mugged by a group of young men of color. This did not lead me to look to police for safety. After all, as I have reviewed in this book, police generally do not reduce crime, clearance rates are low, police act in discriminatory ways, policing perpetuates conditions that produce violence, and "crime" is a term weaponized against the most marginalized.

63 Pride and Joy Families, n.d.

64 Author's field notes, November 2017.

65 Biviano 2019.

66 Author's field notes, January 2019. See Morris 2016.

67 Brown and Schept 2017, 451.

68 Ferrell 2013.

69 As Robin D. G. Kelley (2002, 9) recognizes, "The most radical ideas often grow out of a concrete intellectual engagement with the problems of aggrieved populations confronting systems of oppression."

70 Walter 2019.

71 Author's field notes, August 2017.

72 Rueben Miller (2021, 8) states of the afterlife of mass incarceration, "The prison lives on through the people who've been convicted long after they complete their sentences, and it lives on through the grandmothers, lovers, and children forced to share their burdens because they are never really allowed to pay their so-called debt to society."

73 This is key for what may be called critical pain studies.

74 Purnell 2021, 284–285; Kelley 2002. See McHarris 2024.

APPENDIX

1 Author's field notes, August 2018.

2 Associated Press 2019.

3 Best 2012, 11.

4 Loseke 2003, 28.

5 Formula stories include statements and strategies that, when combined, "create a narrative, a story with a plot and characters, and point of being told" (Loseke 2003, 89). Donileen Loseke (2003, 17) furthermore describes typification "as an image in our heads of typical kinds of things, be these cats, prostitutes, or ecological ruin. Because we cannot know all cats, prostitutes, or instances of environmental ruin, the best we can do is have an image of the *typical*." Key to social problem work is also representation. Stuart Hall (2003, 17) states of representation, "We give things meaning by how we *represent them*—the words we use about them, the stories we tell about them, the images of them we produce, the emotions we associate with them, the ways we classify and conceptualize them, the values we place on them."

6 Hall et al. 1978; Loseke 2003, 59. Erving Goffman (1974, 21) defines a frame as a "schemata of interpretation" that "allows users to locate, perceive, identify, and label a seemingly infinite number of concrete occurrences."

7 Altheide 1997, 651.

8 Walby et al. 2020, 60; Hall 1985.

9 Hartman 2022, 104.

10 Bocock 1986, 33.

11 Bratsis 2016; Gilmore and Gilmore 2008.

12 As Nicos Poulantzas (2014, 17) stated, "The political field of the State (as well as the sphere of ideology) has always, in different forms, been present in the constitution and reproduction of the relations of production."

13 As Nicos Poulantzas (2014, 39) continued, the state "organizes the market and property relations; it institutes political domination and establishes the politically dominant class; and it stamps and codifies all forms of the social division of labour—all social reality—within the framework of a class-divided society."

14 Karl Marx ([1867] 1990, 280) stated that the "free" worker is "someone who has brought his own hide to market and now has nothing to expect—but a tanning." With emancipation, the incorporation of newly freed African Americans, too, was not based on the assertion of rights but the right of contract for indentured servitude (Hartman 2022).

15 Purnell 2021, 261.

16 Michel Foucault (1994, 212) states of subjectification, "There are two meanings of the word *subject*: subject to someone else by control and dependence, and tied to his own identity by a conscience or self-knowledge. Both meanings suggest a form of power which subjugates and makes subject to."

17 Althusser 2014.

18 Linnemann 2016, 17.

19 Correia and Wall 2022, 134.

20 Hall 2003, 8.

21 McKenna 2013.

22 Copes et al. 2023.

23 Miller et al. 2015.

24 Ferrell 2013.

25 Fletcher 2013, 15.

26 Carr 2010, 18.

27 Price 2015a.

28 Sandberg and Copes 2013.

29 Altheide and Schneider 2012.

30 I used the ProQuest digital archival and searched for the keywords "heroin," "opioid," or "opiate" in the *Press & Sun-Gazette* from 2013 to May 2019. This included 85 articles from 2013, 125 articles from 2014, 117 articles from 2015, 266 articles from 2017, 189 articles from 2018, and 48 articles from 2019 until May 24, when my fieldwork ended.

31 Banks 2005; Greer 2007.

32 McClanahan 2021, 119; Mawby 2013.

33 Ferrell and colleagues (2013, 94–99) offer the examples of "trendy clothing displayed in shop windows, commercials marketing transgression, or security cameras littered across public/private spaces."

34 Presdee 2000, 15.

35 Pleus and Revier 2017, 2018; Bush 2018; Perez 2019.

36 The concept of disruptive ethnography emerged out of a conversation with Andrew Pragacz. It was during the spring 2017 "Critical Criminology / Representing Justice" conference held at the University of Ottawa. The event hosted presenters who merged academic and activist practices within a critical criminological framework. Inspired by vibrant discussion, we retired one evening to a local bar in downtown Ottawa to chat. Sipping beer, we reflected on conference themes and our efforts to research *and* address abuses at the local jail—making our engagement disruptive.

37 Goffman 1959, 66; Heritage 2013.
38 Brown and Schept 2017, 454.
39 Schept 2012.
40 Author's field notes, October 2018.
41 Wall and Linnemann 2014.
42 We offered the coordinator a study that showed a decrease in overdose rates in states where cannabis had been legalized (Bachhuber et al. 2014).
43 Author's field notes, March 2019.
44 Arford and Hill 2012.
45 M. Brown 2009. See Revier 2020b, 2021a, 2021b.
46 Hartman 2022, 373.
47 Revier 2022; Punch 2012; Wakeman 2014; Harris 2015.
48 As I recognize in my autoethnographic analysis, I at times utilized terms like "crazy" and "fat" in my field diary, which do reinforce dominant and stigmatizing views of health and well-being. Revier 2022, 324.

REFERENCES

AAMC (Association of American Medical Colleges). 2017. "Healthcare Affects Millions in Rural U.S. Communities." AAMCNews, October 31. https://news.aamc.org.

ABC News. 2010. "The New Face of Heroin Addiction." https://abcnews.go.com.

Abdul-Quader, Abu S., Jonathan Feelemyer, Shilpa Modi, Ellen S. Stein, Alya Briceno, Salaam Semaan, Tara Horvath, Gail E. Kennedy, and Don C. Des Jarlais. 2013. "Effectiveness of Structural-Level Needle/Syringe Programs to Reduce HCV And HIV Infection Among People Who Inject Drugs: A Systematic Review." *AIDS and Behavior* 17:2878–2892.

Abel, Jaison R., and Richard Deitz. 2019. "Why Are Some Places So Much More Unequal than Others? Federal Reserve Bank of New York." *Economic Policy Review* 25 (1).

ABLE (Advocacy, Betterment, Learning, Empowerment). 2025. "ABLE Program Broome County Re-entry." Facebook, February 8. www.facebook.com.

ACLU (American Civil Liberties Union). 2019. "Federal Prison to Provide Medication for Addiction Treatment to Massachusetts Woman." ACLU Massachusetts. June 5. www.aclum.org.

Albany, New York. n.d. "Law Enforcement Assisted Diversion." Accessed February 1, 2025. www.albanyny.gov.

Alexander, Bruce. 2010. *The Globalization of Addiction: A Study in Poverty of the Spirit.* Oxford University Press.

Alexander, Michelle. 2012. *The New Jim Crow: Mass Incarceration in the Age of Colorblindness.* 2nd ed. New Press.

Altheide, David L. 1997. "The News Media, the Problem Frame, and the Production of Fear." *Sociological Quarterly* 38 (4): 647–668.

Altheide, David L. 2003. "Notes Towards a Politics of Fear." *Journal for Crime, Conflict and the Media* 1 (1): 37–54.

Altheide, David L., and Christopher J. Schneider. 2012. *Qualitative Media Analysis.* Sage.

Althusser, Louis. 2014. *On the Reproduction of Capitalism: Ideology and Ideological State Apparatuses.* Verso.

Amsden, David. 2014. "The New Face of Heroin." *Rolling Stone*, April 3. www.rollingstone.com.

Anderson, Ditte. 2015. "Stories of Change in Drug Treatment: A Narrative Analysis of 'Whats' and 'Hows' in Institutional Storytelling." *Sociology of Health & Illness* 37 (5): 668–682.

Anderson, Elijah. 2015. "The White Space." *Sociology of Race and Ethnicity* 1 (1): 10–21.

Anslinger, Harry J., and Courtney R. Cooper. 1937. "Marijuana: Assassin of Youth." *American Magazine* 124 (19).

APA (American Psychiatric Association). 2013. *Diagnostic and Statistical Manual of Mental Disorders.* APA.

Arani, Alexia. 2022. "Abolitionist Care: Crip of Color Worldmaking in the US-Mexico Borderlands." PhD diss., University of California.

Arford, Tammi, and Andrea Hill. 2012. "Role Conflict and Congruence: Academic Sociologists Occupy Boston." *Berkeley Journal of Sociology* 56:132–146.

Armstrong, Sarah. 2018. "The Cell and the Corridor: Imprisonment as Waiting, and Waiting as Mobile." *Time & Society* 27 (2): 133–154.

Arnold, Judy, and Alexis Pleus. 2018. "Women Have No Privacy in Broome County Jail." *Pressconnects*, March 19. www.pressconnects.com.

Arnold, Willis R. 2019. "Setting Precedent, a Federal Court Rules Jail Must Give Inmate Addiction Treatment." National Public Radio, May 4. www.npr.org.

ASAM (American Society of Addiction Medicine). 2017. "Treatment Gap Awareness Week Starts." April 18. www.asam.org.

Asher, Jeff, and Ben Horwitz. 2020. "How Do the Police Actually Spend Their Time?" *New York Times*, June 20. www.nytimes.com.

ASHP (American Social History Project). n.d. "Slave Laws in British Colonial New York, 1664–1731." City University of New York. Accessed January 30, 2025. https://shec.ashp.cuny.edu.

Associated Press. 2019. "Purdue Pharma Considered Profiting Off Treating Those Addicted to Opioids." Telegram, February 1. www.telegram.com.

Aswad, Ed, and Suzanne M. Meredith. 2001. *Binghamton: Images of America.* Arcadia.

Aswad, Ed, and Suzanne M. Meredith. 2005. *IBM: Images of America.* Arcadia.

Athans, Philip. 2014. *Writing Monsters: How to Craft Believably Terrifying Creatures to Enhance Your Horror, Fantasy, and Science Fiction.* Penguin.

Atrens, Dale. 2000. "Drug Addiction as Demonic Possession." *Overland* 158:19–24.

Ayres, Tammy C., and Craig Ancrum. 2023. Introduction to *Understanding Drug Dealing and Illicit Drug Markets: National and International Perspectives*, edited by Tammy C. Ayres and Craig Ancrum. Routledge.

Ayres, Tammy C., and James Treadwell. 2023. "Entrepreneurs: Just Taking Care of Business, the Drug Business." In *Understanding Drug Dealing and Illicit Drug Markets: National and International Perspectives*, edited by Tammy C. Ayres and Craig Ancrum. Routledge.

Bachhuber, Marcus A., Brendan Saloner, Chinazo O. Cunningham, and Colleen L. Barry. 2014. "Medical Cannabis Laws and Opioid Analgesic Overdose Mortality in the United States, 1999–2010." *JAMA Internal Medicine* 174 (10): 1668–1673.

Banks, Mark. 2005. "Spaces of (In)Security: Media and Fear of Crime in a Local Context." *Crime Media Culture* 1 (2): 169–187.

Barnes, Emily. 2021. "Housing Advocates Say Broome's Scarce Options Are 'Putting Households Against Each Other.'" *Pressconnects*, December 15. www.pressconnects.com.

Baum, Dan. 2016. "Legalize It All." *Harper's Magazine*, April 1. https://harpers.org.

Bechteler, Stephane Schmitz, and Kathleen Kane-Willis. 2017. "Whitewashed: The African American Opioid Epidemic." Chicago Urban League, November 1. https://chiul.org.

Becker, Howard S. (1963) 2008. *Outsiders: Studies in the Sociology of Deviance.* Simon and Schuster.

Beckett, Katherine. 2008. "Race and Drug Law Enforcement in Seattle." ACLU Drug Law Reform Project and the Defender Association. www.aclu.org.

Beckett, Katherine. 2014. "Seattle's Law Enforcement Assisted Diversion Program: Lessons Learned from the First Two Years." Unpublished report commissioned by the Ford Foundation. www.researchgate.net.

Beckett, Katherine. 2022. *Ending Mass Incarceration: Why It Persists and How to Achieve Meaningful Reform.* Oxford University Press.

Beckett, Katherine, and Marco Brydolf-Horwitz. 2020. "A Kinder, Gentler Drug War? Race, Drugs, and Punishment in 21st Century America." *Punishment & Society* 22 (4): 509–533.

Belenko, Steven, Nicole Fabrikant, and Nancy Wolff. 2011. "The Long Road to Treatment: Models of Screening and Admission into Drug Courts." *Criminal Justice and Behavior* 38 (12): 1222–1243.

Belenko, Steven, and Cassia Spohn. 2014. *Drugs, Crime, and Justice.* Sage.

Beletsky, Leo. 2019. "America's Favorite Antidote: Drug-Induced Homicide in the Age of Overdose Crisis." SSRN. https://papers.ssrn.com.

Beletsky, Leo, and Corey S. Davis. 2017. "Today's Fentanyl Crisis: Prohibition's Iron Law, Revisited." *International Journal of Drug Policy* 46:156–159.

Bell, Derrick A. 1980. "*Brown v. Board of Education* and the Interest-Convergence Dilemma." *Harvard Law Review* 93 (3): 518–533.

Bell, Michael M. 2007. "The Two-ness of Rural Life and the Ends of Rural Scholarship." *Journal of Rural Studies* 23 (4): 402–415.

Beman, Nathan Sidney Smith. 1829. *Beman on Intemperance: A Discourse Delivered in Stephentown, Dec. 25, 1828, and in Troy, Sabbath Evening, Jan. 11, 1829, Before the Temperance Societies of Those Towns.* J. P. Haven.

Benezet, Anthony. 1778. *Serious Considerations on Several Important Subjects: Viz. on War and Its Inconsistency with the Gospel. Observations on Slavery. And Remarks on the Nature and Bad Effects of Spirituous Liquors.*

Bennett, Hans. 2008. "Organizing to Abolish the Prison-Industrial Complex." *Dissident Voice.* July 11. https://dissidentvoice.org.

Berger, Dan, Mariame Kaba, and David Stein. 2017. "What Abolitionists Do." *Jacobin*, August 24. https://jacobin.com.

Best, Joel. 2012. *Social Problems.* 2nd ed. Norton.

Betty Ford Institute Consensus Panel. 2007. "What Is Recovery? A Working Definition from the Betty Ford Institute." *Journal of Substance Abuse Treatment* 33 (3): 221–228.

Billings. 2017. "LePage in Spotlight for Saying Drug Dealers Impregnate 'White Girls.'" *Press Herald*, November 30. www.pressherald.com.

Bing. n.d. "Shoes Were a Good Fit for Binghamton." Visit Binghamton. Accessed February 2, 2025. https://visitbinghamton.org.

Binghamton Homepage. 2016a. "94-Count Indictment After Biggest Heroin Bust in Broome County History." August 3. www.binghamtonhomepage.com.

Binghamton Homepage. 2016b. "Operation S.A.F.E. Gets Treatment for Addicts." February 8. www.binghamtonhomepage.com.

Binghamton Homepage. 2018. "Broome County Jail Receives State Funding for Jail-Based Substance Abuse Treatment Program." June 29. www.binghamtonhomepage.com.

Binswanger, Ingrid A., Marc F. Stern, Richard A. Deyo, Patrick J. Heagerty, Allen Cheadle, Joann G. Elmore, and Thomas D. Koepsell. 2007. "Release from Prison—A High Risk of Death for Former Inmates." *New England Journal of Medicine* 356 (2): 157–165.

Bisaga, Adam. 2018. *Overcoming Opioid Addiction: The Authoritative Medical Guide for Patients, Families, Doctors, and Therapists.* The Experiment.

Biviano, Ashley. 2018. "With National Focus on Combating Opioid Use, Methamphetamine Deaths Rise in the US." *Press & Sun-Bulletin*, December 2, A6.

Biviano, Ashley. 2019. "Binghamton Residents Protest Alleged Strip Searches of Four Students at East Middle." *Pressconnects*, January 23. www.pressconnects.com.

BJS (Bureau of Justice Statistics). 2009. "Annual Probation Survey and Annual Parole Survey." www.bjs.gov.

Black, Winifred, and Fremont Older. 1928. *Dope: The Story of the Living Dead.* J. J. Little and Ives.

Blackmon, Douglas A. 2009. *Slavery by Another Name: The Re-enslavement of Black Americans from the Civil War to World War II.* Anchor Books.

Blakinger, Keri. 2022. *Corrections in Ink.* St. Martin's.

Bluher, Sarah. 2018. "Law Enforcement Assisted Diversion (LEAD) Is Coming to Ithaca. Who Will It Be For?" *Ithaca Times*, October 23. www.ithaca.com.

Blum, Liz. 2024. "Decarcerating Sacramento: Confronting Jail Expansion in California's Capital." In *The Jail Is Everywhere: Fighting the New Geography of Mass Incarceration*, edited by Jack Norton, Lydia Pelot-Hobbs, and Judah Schept. Verso Books.

BOAC (Broome County Opioid Awareness Council). 2017. "Meeting Minutes." December 1. www.broomecountyny.gov.

BOAC (Broome County Opioid Awareness Council). 2024. "Overdose Prevention Program." Accessed February 20, 2025. www.broomecountyny.gov.

Bocock, Robert. 1986. *Hegemony.* Tavistock Books.

Boivin, Rémi, and Silas Nogueira de Melo. 2023. "Do Police Stations Deter Crime?" *Crime Science* 12 (1): 1–15.

Bonilla-Silva, Eduardo. 2012. "The Invisible Weight of Whiteness: The Racial Grammar of Everyday Life in Contemporary America." *Ethnic and Racial Studies* 35 (2): 173–194.

BOP (US Bureau of Prisons). 2014. "Detoxification of Chemically Dependent Inmates." Clinical Practice Guidelines. www.bop.gov.

BOP (US Bureau of Prisons). 2024. "Offenses." October 19. www.bop.gov.

BOP (US Bureau of Prisons). n.d. "An Overview of the First Step Act." Accessed May 4, 2024. www.bop.gov.

Borrelli, Anthony. 2015a. "DA Candidates Tackle Drug Epidemic in Broome." *Press & Sun-Bulletin*, September 23, A4.

Borrelli, Anthony. 2015b. "Schumer Touts Plan to Aid Broome Police in Drug Fight." *Pressconnects*, April 10. www.pressconnects.com.

Borrelli, Anthony. 2016a. "DA Says 34 Heroin Addicts Sent for Treatment in New Program." *Press & Sun-Bulletin*, March 10, A6.

Borrelli, Anthony. 2016b. "Diversity in the Ranks: City Boosts Police Recruiting." *Pressconnects*, September 27. www.pressconnects.com.

Borrelli, Anthony. 2016c. "Kingpin Case: Man Admits Drug Sale, Faces 8 Years." *Pressconnects*, November 3. www.pressconnects.com.

Borrelli, Anthony. 2016d. "'Kingpin' Case: Woman Pleads Guilty in Drug Trafficking." *Pressconnects*, September 28. www.pressconnects.com.

Borrelli, Anthony. 2016e. "New Drug Court Policy Can Give a Second Chance." *Press & Sun-Bulletin*, February 1, A1.

Borrelli, Anthony. 2016f. "Overdose Deaths: DA's New Investigator to Probe Cases." *Pressconnects*, November 16. www.pressconnects.com.

Borrelli, Anthony. 2016g. "Seven Nabbed in Drug Raids." *Press & Sun-Bulletin*, July 29, A4.

Borrelli, Anthony. 2017a. "Accused Drug Dealer Hid Narcotics in Her Body, Sheriff Says." *Press & Sun-Bulletin*, August 13, A6.

Borrelli, Anthony. 2017b. "Drug Case: Man Sold Heroin to Support Addiction." *Pressconnects*, February 10. www.pressconnects.com.

Borrelli, Anthony. 2017c. "Drug 'Kingpin' Gets 10 Years in State Prison." *Press & Sun-Bulletin*, February 16, A6.

Borrelli, Anthony. 2017d. "Fatal Crash: Driver Impaired by Drugs, Police Say." *Pressconnects*, April 28. www.pressconnects.com.

Borrelli, Anthony. 2017e. "Heroin Dealer Charged in Overdose." *Press & Sun-Bulletin*, September 9, A2.

Borrelli, Anthony. 2017f. "'Top Guy' and 'Bumbling Doofus' Go to Prison." *Pressconnects*, September 8. www.pressconnects.com.

Borrelli, Anthony. 2018a. "Broome DA: Arrested Addicts Can Avoid Prosecution If They Succeed in 90-Day Treatment." *Pressconnects*, July 31. www.pressconnects.com.

Borrelli, Anthony. 2018b. "Broome DA: $281K from Convicted Drug Dealers Will Fund Police, Treatment Efforts." *Pressconnects*, April 26. www.pressconnects.com.

Borrelli, Anthony. 2018c. "Jennifer Grenchus Sentenced to Five Years Probation for Fatal Drugged-Driving Crash." *Pressconnects*, March 16. www.pressconnects.com.

Borrelli, Anthony. 2020a. "Fentanyl Is the Drug Trade's Murderous Menace, and It's Upending Treatment and Policing." *Pressconnects*, December 14. www.pressconnects.com.

Borrelli, Anthony. 2020b. "Thomas Husar Died After His Arrest on a Probation Violation. His Parents Blame the Jail." *Pressconnects*, March 4. www.pressconnects.com.

Borrelli, Anthony, and Jeff Murray. 2017. "Gangs in the Tier: Shooting Cases Have Case a Spotlight." *Pressconnects*, May 12. www.pressconnects.com.

Borrelli, Anthony, and John Roby. 2016. "Addiction Sea Change: Broome DA Vows Help, Not Arrests." *Pressconnects*, February 8. www.pressconnects.com.

Bradford, James. 2021. "The War on Drugs in Afghanistan." In *The War on Drugs: A History*, edited by David Farber. New York University Press.

Bratsis, Peter. 2016. *Everyday Life and the State*. Routledge.

Brecher, E. M. 1972. "How to Launch a Nationwide Drug Menace." In *Consumer Reports Magazine, Licit and Illicit Drugs: The Consumers Union Report on Narcotic Stimulants, Depressants, Inhalants, and Marijuana—Including Caffeine*. Little, Brown.

Bright, Bridget. 2017. "Decarcerate Tompkins County Looks for Its Next Steps." WICB, November 14. https://wicb.org.

Britannica Money. 2024. "IBM." October 22. www.britannica.com.

Broome County. 2017. "Adopted Budget." www.broomecountyny.gov.

Broome County. 2025. "Corrections Division." Accessed June 9, 2025. https://broomecountyny.gov.

Broome County. n.d.-a. "Budgets." Accessed January 30, 2025. www.gobroomecounty.com.

Broome County. n.d.-b. "Probation." Accessed February 8, 2025. www.gobroomecounty.com.

Broome County Office of the Sheriff. 2013. "Inmate Handbook."

Broome County Office of the Sheriff. 2023. "Inmate Handbook."

Brown, Michelle. 2009. *The Culture of Punishment: Prison, Society, and Spectacle*. New York University Press.

Brown, Michelle, and Judah Schept. 2017. "New Abolition, Criminology and a Critical Carceral Studies." *Punishment & Society* 19 (4): 440–462.

Brown, Wendy. 1995. *States of Injury: Power and Freedom in Late Modernity*. Princeton University Press.

Brownstein, Henry H. 1991. "The Media and the Construction of Random Drug Violence." *Social Justice* 18 (4): 85–103.

Buehler, Emily D. 2021. "Sexual Victimization Reported by Adult Correctional Authorities, 2016–2018." US Department of Justice, Bureau of Justice Statistics. https://bjs.ojp.gov.

Bureau of Labor Statistics. 2023. "Economy at a Glance." www.bls.gov.

Burns, Stacy Lee, and Mark Peyrot. 2003. "Tough Love: Nurturing and Coercing Responsibility and Recovery in California Drug Courts." *Social Problems* 50 (3): 416–438.

Burston, Betty Watson, Dionne Jones, and Pat Roberson-Saunders. 1995. "Drug Use and African Americans: Myth Versus Reality." *Journal of Alcohol and Drug Education* 40 (2): 19–39.

Bush, A. J. 2018. "Truth Pharm: Incarceration for Drug Offenses Increases Overdoses." WICZ, January 15. www.wicz.com.

Bush, George H .W. 1990. "Presidential Proclamation 6158." Library of Congress, Project on the Decade of the Brain, July 17. www.loc.gov.

Butler, Judith. 2004. *Precarious Lives: The Powers of Mourning and Violence*. Verso.

Cable, George Washington. 1907. "The Freedman's Case in Equity." In *The Silent South*. Charles Scribner's Sons.

Campbell, Nancy D. 2004. "Technologies of Suspicion: Coercion and Compassion in Post-Disciplinary Surveillance Regimes." *Surveillance & Society* 2 (1): 78–92.

Campbell, Nancy D. 2007. *Discovering Addiction: The Science and Politics of Substance Abuse Research*. University of Michigan Press.

Campbell, Nancy D. 2010. "Toward a Critical Neuroscience of 'Addiction.'" *BioSocieties* 5 (1): 89–104.

Caquet, P. E. 2022. *Opium's Orphans: The 200-Year History of the War on Drugs*. Reaktion Books.

Carr, E. Summerson. 2010. *Scripting Addiction: The Politics of Therapeutic Talk and American Sobriety*. Princeton University Press.

Carroll, Noël. 1990. *The Philosophy of Horror; or, Paradoxes of the Heart*. Routledge.

Case, Anne, and Angus Deaton. 2020. *Deaths of Despair and the Future of Capitalism*. Princeton University Press.

Cavender, Gray, and Mark Fishman. 1998. *Entertaining Crime: Television Reality Programs*. Aldine de Gruyter.

CDC (Centers for Disease Control). 2017a. "Ann Marie." www.cdc.gov.

CDC (Centers for Disease Control). 2017b. "Understanding the Epidemic." www.cdc.gov.

CDC (Centers for Disease Control). 2018. "Drug Overdose Deaths." December 19. www.cdc.gov.

CDC (Centers for Disease Control). 2023. Opioid Overdose. www.cdc.gov.

Census Reporter. 2021. "Broome County, NY (ACS 2021)." August 23. www.censusreporter.org.

CESAR Fax. 2012. "Suboxone Sales Estimated to Reach $1.4 Billion in 2012—More than Viagra or Adderall." Center for Substance Abuse Research, University of Maryland. Vol. 21, no. 49.

Chamayou, Grégoire. 2012. *Manhunts: A Philosophical History*. Princeton University Press.

Chancer, Lynn S. 2010. *High-Profile Crimes*. University of Chicago Press.

Changing the Narrative. n.d. "Fentanyl 'Contact' Overdoses. The Action Lab at the Center for Health Policy and Law. Accessed January 31, 2025. www.changingthenarrative.news.

Chiarello, Elizabeth. 2024. *Policing Patients: Treatment and Surveillance on the Frontlines of the Opioid Crisis*. Princeton University Press.

Christie, Nils. 2007. *The Limits to Pain: The Role of Punishment in Penal Policy*. Wipf and Stock.

Chung, Connie. 2011. *The Politics of (Un)Mothering: A Literature Review on Homeless Mothers*. Lambert.

Churchill, Ward. 2004. *Kill the Indian, Save the Man*. City Lights.

City of Binghamton. n.d. "Finance." Accessed January 30, 2025. www.binghamton-ny.gov.

City of Ithaca. 2016. "The Ithaca Plan: A Public Health and Safety Approach to Drugs and Drug Policy." February. www.cityofithaca.org.

Clifasefi, Seema L., and Susan E. Collins. 2016. "LEAD Program Evaluation: Describing LEAD Case Management in Participants' Own Words." Harm Reduction Research and Treatment Lab, University of Washington, Harborview Medical Center.

Clifasefi, Seema L., Heather S. Lonczak, and Susan E. Collins. 2016. "LEAD Program Evaluation: The Impact of LEAD on Housing, Employment and Income/Benefits." Harm Reduction Research and Treatment Lab, University of Washington, Harborview Medical Center.

Clifasefi, Seema L., Heather S. Lonczak, and Susan E. Collins. 2017. "Seattle's Law Enforcement Assisted Diversion (LEAD) Program: Within-Subjects Changes on Housing, Employment, and Income/Benefits Outcomes and Associations With Recidivism." *Crime & Delinquency* 63 (4): 1–17.

Cobbe, William Rosser. 1985. *Doctor Judas, A Portrayal of the Opium Habit*. Griggs.

Cohen, Peter DA. 2000. "Is the Addiction Doctor the Voodoo Priest of Western Man?" *Addiction Research* 8 (6): 589–598.

Collins, Michael, and Sheila Vakharia. 2020. *Criminal Justice Reform in the Fentanyl Era: One Step Forward, Two Steps Back*. Drug Policy Alliance.

Collins, Susan E., Heather S. Lonczak, and Seema L. Clifasefi. 2015a. "LEAD Program Evaluation: Criminal Justice and Legal System Utilization and Associated Costs." Harm Reduction Research and Treatment Lab, University of Washington, Harborview Medical Center.

Collins, Susan E., Heather S. Lonczak, and Seema L. Clifasefi. 2015b. "LEAD Program Evaluation: Recidivism Report." Harm Reduction Research and Treatment Lab, University of Washington, Harborview Medical Center.

Collins, Susan E., Heather S. Lonczak, and Seema L. Clifasefi. 2017. "Seattle's Law Enforcement Assisted Diversion (LEAD): Program Effects on Recidivism Outcomes." *Evaluation and Program Planning* 64:49–56.

Collins, William J. 1915. "An Address on the Ethics and Law of Drug and Alcohol Addiction." *The Lancet*, October 16.

Columbia University Justice Lab. 2020. "Racial Inequities in New York Parole Supervision." March 12. https://justicelab.columbia.edu.

Confessore, Nicholas. 2012. "Tramps like Them." *New York Times*, February 10. www.nytimes.com.

Congressional Record. 2000. "Drug Addiction Treatment Act of 2000." US Government Publishing Office. www.govinfo.

Connery, Hilary Smith. 2015. "Medication-Assisted Treatment of Opioid Use Disorder: Review of the Evidence and Future Directions." *Harvard Review of Psychiatry* 23 (2): 63–75.

Conrad, Peter. 1992. "Medicalization and Social Control." *Annual Review Sociology* 18 (1):209–232.

Coomber, Ross. 2006. *Pusher Myths: Re-situating the Drug Dealer.* Free Association Books.

Copes, Heith, Sveinung Sandberg, and Jared Ragland. 2023. "Protecting Stories: How Symbolic Boundaries Reduce Victimization and Harmful Drug Use." *Crime & Delinquency* 69 (3): 533–558.

Correia, David, and Tyler Wall. 2022. *Police: A Field Guide.* Verso Books.

Cottler, Linda B., Catina C. O'Leary, Katelin B. Nickel, Jennifer M. Reingle, and Daniel Isom. 2014. "Breaking the Blue Wall of Silence: Risk Factors for Experiencing Police Sexual Misconduct among Female Offenders." *American Journal of Public Health* 104 (2): 338–344.

Council of State Governments Justice Center. 2019. "New Analysis Shows How Parole and Probation Violations Significantly Impact States' Prison Populations and Budgets." Council of State Governments, June 18. https://csgjusticecenter.org.

Courtwright, David T. 2010. "The NIDA Brain Disease Paradigm: History, Resistance and Spinoffs." *BioSocieties* 5 (1): 137–147.

Courtwright, David T. 2019. *The Age of Addiction: How Bad Habits Became Big Business.* Harvard University Press.

Covert, Alyvia. 2017. "Police Prepared to Begin Ithaca LEAD Program with Help of City Resources." *Ithaca Voice*, June 29. https://ithacavoice.com.

Cowles, Colleen. 2019. *War on Us: How the War on Drugs and Myths About Addiction Have Created a War on All of Us.* Fidalgo.

Critical Resistance. 2021. "Reformist Reforms vs. Abolitionist Steps to End Imprisonment." https://criticalresistance.org.

CSPAN. 1986. *Reel America: The World I Never Made. Internet Archive.* December 10.

Current Literature. 1889. "The Female Drug Drunkard: Health in the Household." Vol. 3, pp. 480–481.

Curtin, Mary Ellen. 1992. *Legacies of Struggle: Black Prisoners in the Making of Postbellum Alabama, 1865–1895.* Duke University Press.

Dammer, Harry, and Jay Albanese. 2013. *Comparative Criminal Justice Systems.* 5th ed. Cengage Learning.

Daniels, Jessie. 2012. "Intervention: Reality TV, Whiteness, and Narratives of Addiction." *Critical Perspectives on Addiction* 14:103–125.

Daniels, Jessie, Julie C. Netherland, and Alyssa Patricia Lyons. 2018. "White Women, U.S. Popular Culture, and Narratives of Addiction." *Contemporary Drug Problems* 45 (3): 329–346.

DATA USA. n.d. "Broome County, NY." Accessed February 7, 2025. https://datausa.io.

Davis, Angela Y. 2003. *Are Prisons Obsolete?* Seven Stories.

DEA (US Drug Enforcement Agency). 2016. "DEA Warning to Police and Public: Fentanyl Exposure Kills." US Department of Justice, June 10. www.dea.gov.

DEA (US Drug Enforcement Agency). 2022. "DEA Warns of Brightly-Colored Fentanyl Used to Target Young Americans." www.dea.gov.

DEA (US Drug Enforcement Agency). 2024. "DEA's OD Justice Devotes Critical Resources to Fatal Drug Poisoning and Overdose Death Investigations Across the United States." www.dea.gov.

DeFulio, Anthony, Maxine Stitzer, John Roll, Nancy Petry, Paul Nuzzo, Robert P. Schwartz, and Patricia Stabile. 2013. "Criminal Justice Referral and Incentives in Outpatient Substance Abuse Treatment." *Journal of Substance Abuse Treatment* 45 (1): 70–75.

Degenhardt, Louisa, Jason Grebely, Jack Stone, Matthew Hickman, Peter Vickerman, Brandon D. L. Marshall, Julie Bruneau, Frederick L. Altice, Graeme Henderson, Afarin Rahimi-Movaghar, Sarah Larney. 2019. "Global Patterns of Opioid Use and Dependence: Harms to Populations, Interventions, and Future Action." *The Lancet* 394 (10208): 1560–1579.

Degenhardt, Louisa, Sarah Larney, Jo Kimber, Natasa Gisev, Michael Farrell, Timothy Dobbins, Don J. Weatherburn, Amy Gibson, Richard Mattick, Tony Butler, and Lucy Burns. 2014. "The Impact of Opioid Substitution Therapy on Mortality Post-Release from Prison: Retrospective Data Linkage Study." *Addiction* 109 (8): 1306–1317.

Del Real, Jose A. 2017. "The Bronx's Quiet, Brutal War with Opioids." *New York Times*, October 12. www.nytimes.com.

Delgado, Richard, and Jean Stefancic. 1992. "Images of the Outsider in American Law and Culture: Can Free Expression Remedy Systemic Social Ills." *Cornell Law Review* 77:1258–1297.

Des Jarlais, Don C., Theresa Perlis, Kamyar Arasteh, Lucia V. Torian, Sara Beatrice, Judith Milliken, Donna Mildvan, Stanley Yancovitz, and Samuel R. Friedman. 2005. "HIV Incidence Among Injection Drug Users in New York City, 1990 to 2002: Use of Serologic Test Algorithm to Assess Expansion of HIV Prevention Services." *American Journal of Public Health* 95 (8): 1439–1444.

DHHS (US Department of Health and Human Services). 2024. "Biden-Harris Administration Announces $28 Million in Funding Opportunities for Grants Expanding Treatment Services for Substance Use Disorder." February 2. www.hhs.gov.

Díaz-Cotto, Juanita. 2006. *Chicana Lives and Criminal Justice: Voices from El Barrio.* University of Texas Press.

DOJ (US Department of Justice). 1986. "Anti-Drug Abuse Act of 1986." NCJRS Virtual Library. www.ojp.gov.

DOJ (US Department of Justice). 1994. "Understanding Community Policing: A Framework for Action." Bureau of Justice Assistance. www.ojp.gov.

DOJ (US Department of Justice). 1996. "Justice Department Awards $90 Million to Help States Build More Prison Space and Set Up Drug Testing and Treatment Programs." www.justice.gov.

Donohue, Erin, and Dawn Moore. 2009. "When Is an Offender Not an Offender? Power, the Client and Shifting Penal Subjectivities." *Punishment & Society* 11 (3): 319–336.

DPA (Drug Policy Alliance). 2011. "Drug Courts Are Not the Answer: Toward a Health-Centered Approach to Drug Use." https://drugpolicy.org.

DPA (Drug Policy Alliance). 2017. "An Overdose Death Is Not a Murder: Why Drug-Induced Homicide Are Counterproductive and Inhumane." https://drugpolicy.org.

Du Bois, W. E. B. (1903) 2015. *Souls of Black Folk*. Routledge.

Dubber, Markus D. 2000. "Policing Possession: The War on Crime and the End of Criminal Law." *Journal of Criminal Law & Criminology* 91 (4): 829–996.

Dunbar-Ortiz, Roxanne. 2018. *Loaded: A Disarming History of the Second Amendment*. City Lights Books.

Eaton, Joe. 2017. "King of Boise: The Life and Times of a Teenage Oxycodone Dealer." *Pacific Standard*, November 21. https://psmag.com.

Eaton, William J. 1990. "Disabled Persons Rally, Crawl Up Capitol Steps." *Los Angeles Times*, March 13. www.latimes.com.

Ehlers, Scott. 1999. "Policy Briefing: Asset Forfeiture." Drug Policy Foundation, Washington, DC.

Eife, Erin, and Gabriela Kirk. 2021. "'And You Will Wait . . .': Carceral Transportation in Electronic Monitoring as Part of the Punishment Process." *Punishment & Society* 23 (1): 69–87.

EJI (Equal Justice Initiative). 2017. *Lynching in America: Confronting the Legacy of Racial Terror*. 3rd ed.

Ewing, Eve L. 2019. "Mariame Kaba: Everything Worthwhile Is Done with Other People." *ADI Magazine*. https://adimagazine.com.

Eyre, Eric. 2016. "Drug Firms Poured 780M Painkillers into WV amid Rise of Overdoses." *West Virginia Gazette*, December 17. www.wvgazettemail.com.

Faces of Opioids. n.d. "Faces of Opioids—Stories of Using, Death and Recovery." Facebook. Accessed July 2022. www.facebook.com.

Fagan, Jeffrey, and Richard B. Freeman. 1999. "Crime and Work." *Crime and Justice* 25:225–290.

Fanon, Frantz. 1967. *Black Skin, White Masks*. Grove.

Fatsis, Lambros, and Melayna Lamb. 2022. *Policing the Pandemic: How Public Health Becomes Public Order*. Policy.

Federici, Silvia. 2004. *Caliban and the Witch*. Autonomedia.

Federici, Silvia. 2018. *Witches, Witch-Hunting, and Women*. PM.

Feeley, Malcolm M. 1979. *The Process Is the Punishment: Handling Cases in a Lower Criminal Court*. Russell Sage Foundation.

Feimster, Crystal N. 2022. "Lynching." In *Four Hundred Souls: A Community History of African America, 1619–2019*, edited by Ibram X. Kendi and Keisha N. Blain. One World.

Feinblatt, John, Greg Berman, and Aubrey Fox. 2000. "Institutionalizing Innovation: The New York Drug Court Story." *Fordham Urban Law Journal* 28 (1): 277–292.

Feldman, Allen. 2004. "Deterritorialized Wars of Public Safety." *Social Analysis* 48 (1): 73–80.

Ferrell, Jeff. 2013. "Cultural Criminology and the Politics of Meaning." *Critical Criminology: An International Journal* 21 (3): 257–271.

Ferrell, Jeff, Keith J. Hayward, and Jock Young. 2013. *Cultural Criminology: An Invitation*. 2nd ed. Sage.

Feuer, Alan. 2020. *El Jefe: The Stalking of Chapo Guzman*. Simon and Schuster.

Filter Staff. 2019. "This Groundbreaking Letter from Sheriffs and DAs Calls for MAT in Jails." *Filter*, April 3. https://filtermag.org.

Fisher, Carl E. 2022. *The Urge: Our History of Addiction*. Penguin.

Fleetwood, Jennifer. 2016. "Narrative Habitus: Thinking Through Structure/Agency in the Narratives of Offenders." *Crime Media Culture* 12 (2): 173–192.

Fletcher, Anne M. 2013. *Inside Rehab: The Surprising Truth About Addiction Treatment—and How to Get Help That Works*. Penguin.

Ford, Marlie, and Kevin Revier. 2023. "Social Media Depicts Kensington as 'Zombieland'—And It's Deadly." *Filter*, July 27. https://filtermag.org.

Forman, James. 2012. "Racial Critiques of Mass Incarceration: Beyond the New Jim Crow." *New York University Law Review* 87:101–146.

Forman, James. 2022. "The War on Drugs." In *Four Hundred Souls: A Community History of African America, 1619–2019*, edited by Ibram X. Kendi and Keisha N. Blain. One World.

Foucault, Michel. 1979. "Omnes et Singulatim: Towards a Criticism of Political Reason: The Tanner Lectures on Human Values." Delivered at Stanford University. http://foucault.info.

Foucault, Michel. 1994. "The Ethics of the Concern for the Self as a Practice of Freedom." In *Ethics: Subjectivity and Truth*, edited by Paul Rabinow. Penguin.

Foucault, Michel. 2007. *Security, Territory, Population: Lectures at the Collège de France 1977–1978*. Palgrave Macmillan.

Foucault, Michel. 2010. *The Birth of Biopolitics: Lectures at the Collège de France, 1978–1979*. Picador.

Fox, Katherine. 1999. "Reproducing Criminal Types: Cognitive Treatment for Violent Offenders in Prison." *Sociological Quarterly* 40 (3): 435–453.

Frank, Arthur W. 2010. *Letting Stories Breathe: A Socio-Narratology*. University of Chicago Press.

Frank, David. 2018. "'I Was Not Sick and I Didn't Need to Recover': Methadone Maintenance Treatment (MMT) as a Refuge from Criminalization." *Substance Use & Misuse* 53 (2): 311–322.

Frank, David, Pedro Mateu-Gelabert, David C. Perlman, Suzan M. Walters, Laura Curran, and Honoria Guarino. 2021. "'It's Like 'Liquid Handcuffs': The Effects of Take-Home Dosing Policies on Methadone Maintenance Treatment (MMT) Patients' Lives." *Harm Reduction Journal* 18 (1): 1–10.

Fraser, Suzanne, Adrian Farrugia, and Robyn Dwyer. 2018. "Grievable Lives? Death by Opioid Overdose in Australian Newspaper Coverage." *International Journal of Drug Policy* 59:28–35.

Fraser, Suzanne, David Moore, and Helen Keane. 2014. *Habits: Remaking Addiction*. Palgrave Macmillan.

Friday, Gabreélla. 2022. "Weaponizing and Resisting Time: Race, Gender and Punishment." PhD dissertation, State University of New York at Binghamton.

Friedman, Joseph, Helena Hansen, and Joseph P. Gone. 2023. "What Does the 'Deaths of Despair' Narrative Leave Out?" UCLA Health. www.uclahealth.org.

French, Iris. n.d. "The Broome County Almshouse." Accessed February 1, 2025. https://digitalprojects.binghamton.edu.

Frydl, Kathleen. 2021. "The Pharma Cartel." In *The War on Drugs: A History*, edited by David Farber. New York University Press.

Fuller, Doris, H. Richard Lamb, Michael Biasotti, and John Snook. 2015. "Overlooked in the Undercounted: The Role of Mental Illness in Fatal Law Enforcement Encounters." Office of Research and Public Affairs, Treatment Advocacy Center. www.tac.org.

Gagnon, Daniel. 2021. *A Salem Witch: The Trial, Execution, and Exoneration of Rebecca Nurse*. Westholme.

Garnett, Matthew F., and Arialdi M. Miniño. 2024. "Drug Overdose Deaths in the United States, 2003–2023." *NCHS Data Brief* 522:1–12.

Garriott, William. 2011. *Policing Methamphetamine: Narcopolitics in Rural America*. New York University Press.

Garza, Cristina Rivera. 2020. *Grieving: Dispatches from a Wounded*. Feminist Press at CUNY.

Gelardi, Chris. 2022. "Solitary by Another Name: How State Prisons Are Using 'Therapeutic' Units to Evade Reforms." *New York Focus*, October 5. https://nyfocus.com.

Giblin, Pat. 2023. "Man Charged with Smuggling Drugs into Broome County Jail." *Binghamton Homepage*, April 20. www.binghamtonhomepage.com.

Gill, Nick, Deirdre Conlon, Dominique Moran, and Andrew Burridge. 2018. "Carceral Circuitry: New Directions in Carceral Geography." *Progress in Human Geography* 42 (2): 183–204.

Gilmore, David D. 2009. *Monsters: Evil Beings, Mythical Beasts, and All Manner of Imaginary Terrors*. University of Pennsylvania Press.

Gilmore, Ruth W. 2007. *Golden Gulag: Prisons, Surplus, Crisis, and Opposition in Globalizing California*. University of California Press.

Gilmore, Ruth W. 2015. "The Worrying State of the Abolition Movement." *Social Justice* 23.

Gilmore, Ruth W. 2022. *Abolition Geography: Essays Towards Liberation*. Verso Books.

Gilmore, Ruth W. 2024. Foreword to *The Jail Is Everywhere: Fighting the New Geography of Mass Incarceration*, edited by Jack Norton, Lydia Pelot-Hobbs, and Judah Schept. Verso Books.

Gilmore, Ruth W., and Craig Gilmore. 2008. "Restating the Obvious." In *Indefensible Space: The Architecture of the National Insecurity State*, edited by Michael Sorkin. Routledge.

Gilmore, Ruth, and James Kilgore. 2019. "The Case for Abolition." The Marshall Project, July 19. www.themarshallproject.org.

Go, Julian. 2020. "The Imperial Origins of American Policing: Militarization and Imperial Feedback in the Early 20th Century." *American Journal of Sociology* 125 (5): 1193–1254.

Gobineau, Arthur de. 1915. *The Inequality of Human Races*. G. P. Putnam's Sons.

Godfrey, Dustin. 2023. "Vancouver Activists Rally for DULF Compassion Club after Police Raids." *Filter*, November 6. https://filtermag.org.

Godfrey, Dustin. 2024. "Outpouring of Solidarity as BC Prosecutors Push Back DULF Case." *Filter*, January 17. https://filtermag.org.

Goffman, Erving. 1959. *The Presentation of Self in Everyday Life*. Doubleday.

Goffman, Erving. 1961. *Asylums: Essays on the Social Situation of Mental Patients and Other Inmates*. Anchor Books.

Goffman, Erving. 1974. *Frame Analysis*. Harvard University Press.

Goldstein, Paul J. 1985. "The Drugs/Violence Nexus: A Tripartite Conceptual Framework." *Journal of Drug Issues* 15 (4): 493–506.

Gottschalk, Marie. 2014. *Caught: The Prison State and the Lockdown of American Politics*. Princeton University Press.

Gough, John Bartholomew. 1881. *Sunlight and Shadow*. Worthington.

Goulka, Jeremiah, Valena Elizabeth Beety, Alex Kreit, Anne Boustead, Justine Newman, and Leo Beletsky. 2021. "Drug-Induced Homicide Defense Toolkit." 3rd ed. Health in Justice Action Lab. https://papers.ssrn.com.

Gowan, Teresa, and Sarah Whetstone. 2012. "Making the Criminal Addict: Subjectivity and Social Control in a Strong-Arm Rehab." *Punishment & Society* 14 (1): 69–92.

Greene, Dwight. 1989. "Foreword: Drug Decriminalization: A Chorus in Need of Masterrap's Voice." *Hofstra Law Review* 18 (3): 457–500.

Greene, Jack P. 1987. "The Diary of Colonel Landon Carter of Sabine Hall, 1752–1778 (vol. 2)." Virginia Historical Society.

Greer, Chris. 2007. "News Media, Victims and Crime." In *Victims, Crime, and Society*, edited by Pamela Davies, Peter Francis, and Chris Greer. Sage.

Greer, Chris, and Yvonne Jewkes. 2005. "Extremes of Otherness: Media Images of Social Exclusion." *Social Justice* 32 (1): 20–31.

Grondahl, Paul. 2014. "How Heroin Claimed the Life of a Cop's Daughter." *Times Union*, October 27. www.timesunion.com.

Guest Contributor. 2017. "Opinion: New Cortland County Jail Facility Is Not the Solution." *Cortland Voice*, December 12. https://cortlandvoice.com.

Gumbs, Alexis Pauline. 2023. "Learning to Listen." In *Healing Justice Lineages: Dreaming at the Crossroads of Liberation, Collective Care, and Safety*, edited by Cara Page and Erica Woodland. North Atlantic Books.

Gusfield, Joseph R. 1986. *Symbolic Crusade: Status Politics and the American Temperance Movement*. 2nd ed. Urbana: University of Illinois Press.

Hadden, Sally E. 2003. *Slave Patrols: Law and Violence in Virginia and the Carolinas*. Harvard University Press.

Hall, Stuart. 1985. "Signification, Representation, Ideology: Althusser and the Post-Structuralist Debates." *Critical Studies in Media Communication* 2 (2): 91–114.

Hall, Stuart. 2003. Introduction to *Representation: Cultural Representations and Signifying Practices*, edited by Stuart Hall. Sage.

Hall, Stuart, Chas Critcher, Tony Jefferson, John Clarke, and Brian Roberts. 1978. *Policing the Crisis: Mugging, the State, and Law and Order*. Holmes and Meier.

Halushka, John M. 2020. "The Runaround: Punishment, Welfare, and Poverty Survival After Prison." *Social Problems* 67 (2): 233–250.

Hamilton, Leah, Corey S. Davis, Nicole Kravitz-Wirtz, William Ponicki, and Magdalena Cerdá. 2021. "Good Samaritan Laws and Overdose Mortality in the United States in the Fentanyl Era." *International Journal of Drug Policy* 97:103294.

Hamilton Project. 2016. "Rates of Drug Use and Sales, by Race; Rates of Drug Related Criminal Justice Measures by Race." October 20. www.hamiltonproject.org.

Hampton, Ryan. 2024. *Fentanyl Nation: Toxic Politics and America's Failed War on Drugs*. St. Martin's.

Haney-López, Ian F. 2006. *White by Law: The Legal Construction of Race*. 2nd ed. New York University Press.

Hansen, Helena. 2017. "Assisted Technologies of Social Reproduction: Pharmaceutical Prosthesis for Gender, Race, and Class in the White Opioid 'Crisis.'" *Contemporary Drug Problems* 44 (4): 321–338.

Hansen, Helena. 2023. "Pharmakon of Racial Poisons and Cures." In *Whiteout: How Racial Capitalism Changed the Color of Opioids in America*, edited by Helena Hansen, Jules Netherland, and David Herzberg. University of California Press.

Hansen, Helena, Jules Netherland, and David Herzberg. 2023a. "How to See Whiteness." In *Whiteout: How Racial Capitalism Changed the Color of Opioids in America*, edited by Helena Hansen, Jules Netherland, and David Herzberg. University of California Press.

Hansen, Helena, Jules Netherland, and David Herzberg. 2023b. "OxyContin's Racial Precision." In *Whiteout: How Racial Capitalism Changed the Color of Opioids in America*, edited by Helena Hansen, Jules Netherland, and David Herzberg. University of California Press.

Hari, Johann. 2015. *Chasing the Scream: The First and Last Days of the War on Drugs*. Bloomsbury.

Harocopos, Alex, Brent E. Gibson, Nilova Saha, Michael T. McRae, Kailin See, Sam Rivera, and Dave A. Chokshi. 2022. "First 2 Months of Operation at First Publicly Recognized Overdose Prevention Centers in US." *JAMA Network Open* 5 (7): e2222149.

Harriet Tubman Collective. 2017. "Disability Solidarity: Completing the Vision for Black Lives." *Harvard Journal of African American Public Policy*, 69–72.

Harris, Magdalena. 2015. "'Three in the Room': Embodiment, Disclosure, and Vulnerability in Qualitative Research." *Qualitative Health Research* 25 (12): 1689–1699.

Hart, Carl. 2013. *High Price: A Neuroscientist's Journey of Self-Discovery That Challenges Everything You Know About Drugs and Society*. HarperCollins.

Hart, Carl. 2021. *Drug Use for Grown-Ups: Chasing Liberty in the Land of Fear*. Penguin.

Hartman, Saidiya. 2022. *Scenes of Subjection: Terror, Slavery, and Self-Making in Nineteenth-Century America*. 2nd ed. Norton.

Harvard Mental Health Letter. 2011. "How Addiction Hijacks the Brain." July. www.health.harvard.edu.

Harvey, David. 2007. *A Brief History of Neoliberalism*. Oxford University Press.

Harvey, David. 2012. *Rebel Cities: From the Right to the City to the Urban Revolution.* Verso.

Harvey, David. 2017. *Marx, Capital, and the Madness of Economic Reason.* Oxford University Press.

Hassan, Jude. 2012. *Suburban Junkie: From Honor Role, to Heroin Addict.* Mill City.

Hassan, Shira. 2023. "Holding Our Beautiful Mess: Liberatory Harm Reduction and Our Right to Heal." In *Healing Justice Lineages: Dreaming at the Crossroads of Liberation, Collective Care, and Safety,* edited by Cara Page and Erica Woodland. North Atlantic Books.

Hay, James, Stuart Hall, and Lawrence Grossberg. 2013. "Interview with Stuart Hall." *Communication and Critical/Cultural Studies* 10 (1): 10–33.

Hayes, Kelly E. 2022. "Ruth Wilson Gilmore on Abolition, the Climate Crisis, and What Must Be Done." *Truthout,* April 14. https://truthout.org.

Hayes, Kelly E., and Mariame Kaba. 2023. *Let This Radicalize You: Organizing and the Revolution of Reciprocal Care.* Haymarket Books.

Hazlitt, S. 2016. "Levchak, 26-Year-Old, Killed by Heroin, Was a Gentle Soul." *Press & Sun-Bulletin,* March 24, A7.

Health in Justice. 2020. "Drug-Induced Homicide." Action Lab. www.healthinjustice.org.

Helepololei, Justin. 2024. "Against Care: Abolition and the Progressive Jail Assemblage." *Studies in Social Justice* 18 (2): 283–303.

Helling, Steve, and Alexandra Rockey Flemming. 2017. "Faces of an Epidemic." *People,* August 9. https://people.com.

Henrichson, Christian, Jacob Kang-Brown, and Oliver Hinds. 2018. "Expanding Our Knowledge on Local Incarceration Trends." Vera Institute of Justice, December 13. www.vera.org.

Herb, Joshua N., Brittney M. Williams, Kevin A. Chen, Jessica C. Young, Brooke A. Chidgey, Peggy P. McNaull, and Karyn B. Stitzenberg. 2021. "The Impact of Standard Postoperative Opioid Prescribing Guidelines on Racial Differences in Opioid Prescribing: A Retrospective Review." *Surgery* 170 (1): 180–185.

Heritage, John. 2013. *Garfinkel and Ethnomethodology.* Wiley.

Herzberg, David. 2021. "Between the Free Market and the Drug War." In *The War on Drugs: A History,* edited by David Farber. New York University Press.

Herzberg, David. 2023. "'Mother's Little Helpers': White Narcotics in the Medicine Cabinet." In *Whiteout: How Racial Capitalism Changed the Color of Opioids in America,* edited by Helena Hansen, Jules Netherland, and David Herzberg. University of California Press.

Herzing, Rachel. 2015. "Big Dreams and Bold Steps Toward a Police-Free Future." *Truthout,* September 16. https://truthout.org.

Hickman, Timothy A. 2000. "Drugs and Race in American Culture: Orientalism in the Turn-of-the-Century Discourse of Narcotic Addiction." *American Studies* 40 (1): 71–91.

Higginbotham, A. Leon, Jr. 1989. "Race, Sex, Education and Missouri Jurisprudence: Shelley v. Kraemer in a Historical Perspective." *Washington University Law Quarterly* 67 (3): 673–708.

Hinton, Elizabeth, and DeAnza Cook. 2021. "The Mass Criminalization of Black Americans: A Historical Overview." *Annual Review of Criminology* 4 (1): 261–286.

Hobbes, Thomas. (1651) 1982. *Leviathan*. Penguin.

Holland, Sharon Patricia. 2000. *Raising the Dead: Readings of Death and (Black) Subjectivity*. Duke University Press.

hooks, bell. 1992. *Black Looks: Race and Representation*. South End.

hooks, bell. 2004. *The Will to Change: Men, Masculinity, and Love*. Washington Square Press.

hooks, bell. 2006. *Outlaw Cultures: Resisting Representations*. Routledge.

hooks, bell. 2012. *Writing Beyond Race*. Routledge.

Ingraham, Cristopher. 2014. "White People Are More Likely to Deal Drugs, but Black People Are More Likely to Get Arrested for It." *Washington Post*, September 30. www.washingtonpost.com.

Irwin, John. (1985) 2013. *The Jail: Managing the Underclass in American Society*. University of California Press.

Isenberg, Nancy. 2016. *White Trash: The 400-Year Untold History of Class in America*. Penguin.

Jackson, Angie. 2019. "She Died of Opioid Withdrawal in SC Jail Custody: Family Wants Officials Held Accountable." *Post and Courier*, May 24. www.postandcourier.com.

Jacobs, Harrison. 2016. "Here's Why Opioid Epidemic So Bad in West Virginia." *Business Insider*, May 1. www.businessinsider.com.

James, Keturah, and Ayana Jordan. 2018. "The Opioid Crisis in Black Communities." *Journal of Law, Medicine & Ethics* 46 (2): 404–421.

Jarvis, Margaret, Jessica Williams, Matthew Hurford, Dawn Lindsay, Piper Lincoln, Leila Giles, Peter Luongo, and Taleen Safarian. 2017. "Appropriate Use of Drug Testing in Clinical Addiction Medicine." *Journal of Addiction Medicine* 11 (3): 163–173.

Jeffreys, Derek. 2018. *America's Jails: The Search for Human Dignity in an Age of Mass Incarceration*. New York University Press.

Jellinek, E. M. 1960. *The Disease Conception of Alcoholism*. Hillhouse.

Jenkins, Philip. 1994. "'The Ice Age': The Social Construction of a Drug Panic." *Justice Quarterly* 11 (1):7–31.

Jenkins, Philip. 1999. *Synthetic Panics: The Symbolic Politics of Designer Drugs*. New York University Press.

Johnson, Walter. 2001. *Soul by Soul: Life Inside the Antebellum Slave Market*. Harvard University Press.

Johnston, Peg. 2018. "PLOT: Progressive Leaders of Tomorrow." *The Bridge: Binghamton's Community Link*, August 10. https://binghamtonbridge.org.

Joseph, Bob. 2016. "Broome County DA Uses Billboards to Address Drug Dealers." *WNBF*, June 28. https://wnbf.com.

JUST (Justice and Unity for the Southern Tier). 2022. "Sheriff Harder Loses Major Lawsuit JUST and Families Celebrate the Return to In-Person Visitation." May 13. www.justicest.com.

Kaba, Mariame. 2014. "Police 'Reforms' You Should Always Oppose." *Truthout*, December 7. https://truthout.org.

Kaba, Mariame. 2017. "Free Us All—Participatory Defense Campaigns as Abolitionist Organizing." *Agency*, May 8. www.anarchistagency.com.

Kaba, Mariame. 2018. "Circles of Grief, Circles of Healing." In *The Long Term: Resisting Life Sentences, Working Toward Freedom*, edited by Alice Kim, Erica R. Meiners, Audrey Petty, Jill Petty, Beth E. Richie, and Sarah Ross. Haymarket Books.

Kaba, Mariame. 2020. "So You're Thinking About Becoming an Abolitionist." *Medium*, October 30. https://level.medium.com.

Kaba, Mariame, and Kelly Hayes. 2018. "A Jailbreak of the Imagination: Seeing Prisons for What They Are and Demanding Transformation." *Truthout*, May 3. https://truthout.org.

Kaba, Mariame, and Andrea J. Ritchie. 2022. *No More Police: A Case for Abolition*. New Press.

Kaczynski, Andrew. 2019. "Biden in 1993 Speech Pushing Crime Bill Warned of Predators on Our Streets' Who Were 'Beyond the Pale.'" *CNN*, March 7. www.cnn.com.

Kaeble, Danielle. 2023. *Probation and Parole in the United States, 2021*. Bureau of Justice Statistics. https://bjs.ojp.gov.

Kappeler, Victor E., and Gary W. Potter. 2017. *The Mythology of Crime and Criminal Justice*. Waveland.

Karshner, Edward L. 2019. "The Stories Sustain Me: The WYRD-ness of My Appalachia." In *Appalachian Reckoning: A Region Responds to Hillbilly Elegy*, edited by Meredith McCarroll and Anthony Harkins. West Virginia University Press.

Katz, Josh, and Margot Sanger-Katz. 2018. "'The Numbers Are So Staggering.' Overdose Deaths Set a Record Last Year." *New York Times*, November 29. www.nytimes.com.

Kavanaugh, Philip R. 2022. "Narcan as Biomedical Panic: The War on Overdose and the Harms of Harm Reduction." *Theoretical Criminology* 26 (1): 132–152.

Kaye, Kerwin. 2019. *Enforcing Freedom: Drug Courts, Therapeutic Communities, and the Intimacies of the State*. Columbia University Press.

Keane, Helen. 2002. *What's Wrong with Addiction?* Melbourne University Press.

Kelley, Robin D. G. 2002. *Freedom Dreams: The Black Radical Imagination*. Beacon.

Kellogg, John Harvey. 1907. "A Ban on Rum in the South: To Save the Negro from Bestiality the White Men of the Southern States Are Becoming Sober Themselves." *Good Health* 42:522.

Kendi, Ibram X. 2016. *Stamped from the Beginning: The Definitive History of Racist Ideas in America*. Bold Type Books.

Kilgore, James. 2014. "Repackaging Mass Incarceration." *Counterpunch*. www.counterpunch.org.

Kilgore, James. 2022. *Understanding E-Carceration: Electronic Monitoring, the Surveillance State, and the Future of Mass Incarceration*. New Press.

Kim, Jaeok, Quinn Hood, and Elliot Connors. 2021. "The Impact of New York Bail Reform on Statewide Jail Populations: A First Look." Vera: Institute of Justice. www.vera.org.

King, Timothy McMahan. 2019. *Addiction Nation: What the Opioid Crisis Reveals About Us*. Menno Media.

Klein, Andrew R., and Jessica L. Klein. 2022. *Death Before Sentencing: Ending Rampant Suicide, Overdoses, Brutality, and Malpractice in America's Jails*. Rowman and Littlefield.

Klinger, David. 2012. "Dealing with Downed Suspects: Some Lessons from the VALOR Project About How to Properly Manage the Immediate Aftermath of Officer-Involved Shootings." *Police Chief* 79 (5): 24–29.

Knipe, Ed. 1995. *Culture, Society, and Drugs: The Social Science Approach to Drug Use*. Waveland.

Kohler-Hausmann, Julilly. 2010. "'The Attila the Hun Law': New York's Rockefeller Drug Laws and the Making of a Punitive State." *Journal of Social History* 44 (1): 71–95.

Kruis, Nathan E., Katherine McLean, Payton Perry, and Marielle K. Nackley. 2022. "First Responders' Views of Naloxone: Does Stigma Matter?" *Substance Use & Misuse* 57 (10): 1534–1544.

Krupanski, Marc. 2017. "It's Time to Kick Our Addiction to the War On Drugs." *Stat News*, April 25. www.statnews.com.

Kuhns, Joseph B., Kristie R. Blevins, and Seungmug "Zech" Lee. 2012. "Understanding Decisions to Burglarize from the Offender's Perspective." University of North Carolina at Charlotte, Department of Criminal Justice & Criminology.

Kushner, Rachel. 2019. "Is Prison Necessary? Ruth Wilson Gilmore Might Change Your Mind." *New York Times*, April 17. www.nytimes.com.

Lagisetty, Pooja A., Ryan Ross, Amy Bohnert, Michael Clay, and Donovan T. Maust. 2019. "Buprenorphine Treatment Divide by Race/Ethnicity and Payment." *JAMA Psychiatry* 76 (9): 979–981.

Lassiter, Matthew D. 2023. *The Suburban Crisis: White America and the War on Drugs*. Princeton University Press.

Law, John. 2009. "Collateral Realities." Heterogeneities.net. www.heterogeneities.net.

Law, Victoria. 2015. "U.S. Prisons and Jails Are Threatening the Lives of Pregnant Women and Babies." *In These Times*, September 28. https://inthesetimes.com.

Law, Victoria. 2021. *"Prisons Make Us Safer": And 20 Other Myths About Mass Incarceration*. Beacon.

Lawrence, Charles R. 1987. "The Id, the Ego, and Equal Protection: Reckoning with Unconscious Racism." *Stanford Law Review* 39 (2): 235–257.

Lazarus, Jeffrey V., Kelly Safreed-Harmon, Kristina L. Hetherington, Daniel J. Bromberg, Denise Ocampo, Niels Graf, Anna Dichtl, Heino Stöver, and Hans Wolff. 2018. "Health Outcomes for Clients of Needle and Syringe Programs in Prisons." *Epidemiologic Reviews* 40 (1): 96–104.

LEAD. 2017a. "Core Principles for Policing Role." National Support Bureau. January 6. www.leadbureau.org.

LEAD. 2017b. "Core Principles for Prosecutor Role." January 6. www.leadbureau.org.

LEAD. 2020a. "Core Principles for Policing Role." April 3. www.leadbureau.org.

LEAD. 2020b. "Core Principles for Prosecutor Role." April 3. www.leadbureau.org.

LEAD. n.d. "LEAD Sites." National Support Bureau. Accessed February 1, 2025. www.leadbureau.org.

Leas, Emily. 2017. "The Faces of Opioid Addiction." *Brava*, May 1. https://bravamagazine.com.

Lee, Jonathan. 2013. "The New Face of Drug Addiction." *Fox News*, July 19. http://fox40.com.

Lembke, Anna. 2021. *Dopamine Nation: Finding Balance in the Age of Indulgence*. Penguin.

Leshner, Alan I. 1997. "Addiction Is a Brain Disease. And It Matters." *Science* 278 (5335): 45–47.

Levine, Harry G. 1978. "The Discovery of Addiction: Changing Conceptions of Habitual Drunkenness in America." *Journal of Studies on Alcohol* 39 (1): 143–174.

Lewis, Talila A. 2021. "Disability Justice Is an Essential Part of Abolishing Police & Ending Incarceration." In *Abolition for the People: The Movement for a Future Without Policing and Prisons*, edited by Colin Kaepernick. Haymarket Books.

LII (Legal Information Institute). 2022. "Decriminalization." September. www.law.cornell.edu.

Lilley, David R. 2017. "Did Drug Courts Lead to Increased Arrest and Punishment of Minor Drug Offenses?" *Justice Quarterly* 34 (4): 674–698.

Lilley, David R., Kristen DeVall, and Kasey Tucker-Gail. 2019. "Drug Courts and Arrest for Substance Possession: Was the African American Community Differentially Impacted?" *Crime & Delinquency* 65 (3): 352–374.

Lilley, David R., Megan C. Stewart, and Kasey Tucker-Gail. 2020. "Drug Courts and Net-Widening in US Cities: A Reanalysis Using Propensity Score Matching." *Criminal Justice Policy Review* 31 (2): 287–308.

Lim, Sungwoo, Amber L. Seligson, Farah M. Parvez, Charles W. Luther, Maushumi P. Mavinkurve, Ingrid A. Binswanger, and Bonnie D. Kerker. 2012. "Risks of Drug-Related Death, Suicide, and Homicide During the Immediate Post Release Period Among People Released from New York City Jails, 2001–2005." *American Journal of Epidemiology* 175 (6): 519–526.

Link, Bruce G., and Jo C. Phelan. 2001. "Conceptualizing Stigma." *Annual Review of Sociology* 27 (1): 363–385.

Linnemann, Travis. 2016. *Meth Wars: Police, Media, Power*. New York University Press.

Linnemann, Travis. 2017. "Proof of Death: Police Power and the Visual Economies of Seizure, Accumulation and Trophy." *Theoretical Criminology* 21 (1): 57–77.

Linnemann, Travis. 2022. *The Horror of Police*. University of Minnesota Press.

Linnemann, Travis, and Corina Medley. 2023. "Side Affects May Vary: Palliative Capitalism, Punitive Capitalism and US Consumer Culture." In *Understanding Drug Dealing and Illicit Drug Markets: National and International Perspectives*, edited by Tammy C. Ayres and Craig Ancrum. Routledge.

Linnemann, Travis, and Tyler Wall. 2013. "'This Is Your Face on Meth': The Punitive Spectacle of 'White Trash' in the Rural War on Drugs." *Theoretical Criminology* 17 (3): 315–334.

Linnemann, Travis, Tyler Wall, and Edward Green. 2014. "The Walking Dead and Killing State: Zombification and the Normalization of Police Violence." *Theoretical Criminology* 18 (4): 506–527.

Lipsitz, George. 2007. "The Racialization of Space and the Spatialization of Race: Theorizing the Hidden Architecture of Landscape." *Landscape Journal* 26 (1): 10–23.

Loader, Ian. 1997. "Policing and the Social: Questions of Symbolic Power." *British Journal of Sociology* 48 (1): 1–18.

Locke, John. (1689) 1980. *Second Treatise of Government*. Hackett.

Long, Carolyn Morrow. 2007. *A New Orleans Voudou Priestess: The Legend and Reality of Marie Laveau*. University Press of Florida.

Lopez, German. 2019. "A New Study Shows America's Drug Overdose Crisis Is by Far the Worst Among Wealthy Countries." *Vox*, February 26. www.vox.com.

Loseke, Donileen. 2003. *Thinking About Social Problems: An Introduction to Constructionist Perspectives*. 2nd ed. Aldine Transactions.

Lubben, Alex. 2023. "Workers Blame Low Pay and Understaffing for New York's Benefits Backlog." *New York Focus*, June 5. https://nyfocus.com.

Lupick, Travis. 2022. *Light Up The Night: America's Overdose Crisis and the Drug Users Fighting for Survival*. New Press.

Macy, Beth. 2012a. "The Damage Done: Getting Addicted." *Roanoke Times*, September 2. https://roanoke.com.

Macy, Beth. 2012b. "The Damage Done: Heroin Hits Home." *Roanoke Times*, September 3. https://roanoke.com.

Macy, Beth. 2018. *Dopesick: Dealers, Doctors, and the Drug Company That Addicted America*. Little, Brown.

Macy, Beth. 2022. *Raising Lazarus: Hope, Justice, and the Future of America's Overdose Crisis*. Little, Brown.

Madison, Samantha. 2019. "Brindisi: Fund Border Patrol to Stop Fentanyl." *Utica (NY) Observer-Dispatch*, April 1. www.uticaod.com.

Malm, Aili, Dina Perrone, and Erica Magaña. 2020. "Law Enforcement Assisted Diversion (LEAD) External Evaluation." Report to the California State Legislature.

Mancuso, Peter A. 2010. "Resentencing After the 'Fall' of Rockefeller: The Failure of the Drug Law Reform Acts of 2004 and 2005 to Remedy the Injustices of New York's Rockefeller Drug Laws and the Compromise of 2009." *Albany Law Review* 73 (4): 1536–1581.

Manderson, Desmond. 2005. "Possessed: Drug Policy, Witchcraft and Belief." *Cultural Studies* 19 (1): 35–62.

Manjapra, Kris. 2022. *Black Ghost of Empire: The Long Death of Slavery and the Failure of Emancipation*. Simon and Schuster.

Mars, Sarah G., Philippe Bourgois, George Karandinos, Fernando Montero, and Daniel Ciccarone. 2014. "'Every "Never" I Ever Said Came True': Transitions from Opioid Pills to Heroin Injecting." *International Journal of Drug Policy* 25 (2): 257–266.

Marshall, Brandon D. L., Michael Jay Milloy, Evan Wood, Julio S. G. Montaner, and Thomas Kerr. 2011. "Reduction in Overdose Mortality after the Opening of North

America's First Medically Supervised Safer Injecting Facility: A Retrospective Population-Based Study." *The Lancet* 377 (9775): 1429–1437.

Martin, Bill. 2014. "Militarized Police Escalate Conflicts." *Pressconnects*, August 28. www.pressconnects.com.

Martin, Bill. 2018. "Whose [*sic*] White at the BC Jail? We Don't Know?" *Just Talk*, September 14. https://justtalk.blog.

Martin, Bill. 2019a. "Rob Card's Death: 'Broome County Is Killing Me.'" *Just Talk*, March 12. https://justtalk.blog.

Martin, Bill. 2019b. "Stealing from the Families of the Incarcerated." *Just Talk*, May 8. https://justtalk.blog.

Martin, Bill. 2020. "Defunding the Police & Sheriff." *Just Talk*, June 10. https://justtalk.blog.

Martin, Bill. 2022a. "Broome County Jail's Secret $ Millions: Profiting from COVID and Incarcerated Families." *Just Talk*, June 3. https://justtalk.blog.

Martin, Bill. 2022b. "Got a Grievance About Abuse Today? Tomorrow? Ever? Not in the BC Jail You Don't!" *Just Talk*, March 26. https://justtalk.blog.

Martin, Bill. 2022c. "What Does July 4 Mean to Bingham's Town? Slavery and Binghamton Retold." *Just Talk*, January 13. https://justtalk.blog.

Martin, Bill. 2024. "In NY Jails, Prisoners Must Submit Their Abuse Grievances to Their Abusers." *Truthout*, March 24. https://truthout.org.

Marton, Anita, and Gabrielle de la Guéronnière. 2019. "Recent Court Actions Impacting the Substance Use and Disorder Field." Legal Action Center. https://nasadad.org.

Marx, Karl. 1844. "On the Jewish Question." *Works of Karl Marx 1844*. www.marxists.org.

Marx, Karl. (1867) 1990. *Capital: A Critique of Political Economy*. Vol. 1. Penguin.

Massing, Michael. 1998. *The Fix*. Simon and Schuster.

Maté, Gabor. 2008. *In the Realm of Hungry Ghosts: Close Encounters with Addiction*. Random House.

Matsuda, Mari J. 1989. "When the First Quail Calls: Multiple Consciousness as Jurisprudential Method." *Women's Rights Law Reporter* 11:7–10.

Mattlin, Ben. 2022. *Disability Pride: Dispatches from a Post-ADA World*. Beacon.

Mawby, Rob. 2013. *Policing Images*. Willan.

Mbembe, Joseph-Achille. 2019. *Necropolitics*. Duke University Press.

McClanahan, Bill. 2021. *Visual Criminology*. Policy.

McClellan, Chandler, Barrot H. Lambdin, Mir M. Ali, Ryan Mutter, Corey S. Davis, Eliza Wheeler, Michael Pemberton, and Alex H. Kral. 2018. "Opioid-Overdose Laws Association with Opioid Use and Overdose Mortality." *Addictive Behaviors* 86:90–95.

McHarris, Philip V. 2024. *Beyond Policing*. Hachette UK.

McKean, Jerome, and Kiesha Warren-Gordon. 2011. "Racial Differences in Graduation Rates from Adult Drug Treatment Courts." *Journal of Ethnicity in Criminal Justice* 9 (1): 41–55.

McKenna, Stacey. 2013. "The Meth Factor: Stigma, Authoritative Discourse, and Women Who Use." *Contemporary Drug Problems* 40 (3): 351–385.

McKim, Allison. 2017. *Addicted to Rehab: Race, Gender, and Drugs in the Era of Mass Incarceration.* Rutgers University Press.

McLellan, A. Thomas, David C. Lewis, Charles P. O'Brien, and Herbert D. Kleber. 2000. "Drug Dependence, a Chronic Medical Illness: Implications for Treatment, Insurance, and Outcomes Evaluation." *Journal of the American Medical Association* 284 (13): 1689–1695.

McQuade, Brendan. 2020. "The Prose of Pacification: Critical Theory, Police Power, and Abolition Socialism." *Social Justice* 47 (3–4): 55–76.

McQuade, Brenden, and Mark Neocleous. 2020. "Beware: Medical Police." *Radical Philosophy* 2 (4): 3–9.

Medical and Surgical Reporter. 1887. "The Opium Habit in San Francisco." December 10.

Meghani, Salimah H., Eeseung Byun, and Rollin M. Gallagher. 2012. "Time to Take Stock: A Meta-Analysis and Systematic Review of Analgesic Treatment Disparities for Pain in the United States." *Pain Medicine* 13 (2):150–174.

Merrall, Elizabeth L. C., Azar Kariminia, Ingrid A. Binswanger, Michael S. Hobbs, Michael Farrell, John Marsden, Sharon J. Hutchinson, and Sheila M. Bird. 2010. "Meta-Analysis of Drug-Related Deaths Soon After Release from Prison." *Addiction* 105 (9): 1545–1554.

Métraux, Alfred. 1959. *Voodoo in Haiti.* Pickle Partners.

Metzl, Jonathan M. 2024. *Dying of Whiteness: How the Politics of Racial Resentment is Killing America's Heartland.* Basic Books.

Michaud, Liam, and Emily van der Meulen. 2023. "'They're Just Watching You All the Time': The Surveillance Web of Prison Needle Exchange." *Surveillance & Society* 21 (2): 154–170.

Miles, Tiya. 2015. *Tales from the Haunted South: Dark Tourism and Memories of Slavery from the Civil War Era.* University of North Carolina Press.

Miller, Jody, Kristin Carbone-Lopez, and Mikh V. Gunderman. 2015. "Gendered Narratives of Self, Addiction, and Recovery Among Women Methamphetamine Users." In *Narrative Criminology: Understanding Stories of Crime,* edited by Lois Presser and Sveinung Sandberg. New York University Press.

Miller, Reuben J. 2014. "Devolving the Carceral State: Race, Prisoner Reentry, and the Micro-Politics of Urban Poverty Management." *Punishment & Society* 16 (3): 305–335.

Miller, Reuben J. 2021. *Halfway Home: Race, Punishment, and the Afterlife of Mass Incarceration.* Little, Brown.

Miller, Reuben J., and Forrest Stuart. 2017. "Carceral Citizenship: Race, Rights and Responsibility in the Age of Mass Supervision." *Theoretical Criminology* 21 (4): 532–548.

Mills, C. Wright. 1940. "Situated Actions and Vocabularies of Motive." *American Sociological Review* 5 (6): 904–913.

Milstein, Cindy. 2017. "Prologue: Cracks in the Wall." *Rebellious Mourning: The Collective Work of Grief*, edited by Cindy Milstein. AK Press.

Mitchell, Ojmarrh, David B. Wilson, Amy Eggers, and Doris L. MacKenzie. 2012. "Assessing the Effectiveness of Drug Courts on Recidivism: A Meta-Analytic Review of Traditional and Non-Traditional Drug Courts." *Journal of Criminal Justice* 40 (1): 60–71.

Mohamed, A. Rafik, and Erik D. Fritsvold. 2009. *Dorm Room Dealers: Drugs and the Privileges of Race and Class*. Lynne Rienner.

Moore, David, and Suzanne Fraser. 2013. "Producing the 'Problem' of Addiction in Drug Treatment." *Qualitative Health Research* 23 (7): 916–923.

Moore, Dawn. 2007. "Translating Justice and Therapy: The Drug Treatment Court Networks." *British Journal of Criminology* 47 (1): 42–60.

Moore, Dawn. 2011. "The Benevolent Watch: Therapeutic Surveillance in Drug Treatment Court." *Theoretical Criminology* 15 (3): 255–268.

Moore, Dawn, Lisa Freeman, and Marian Krawczyk. 2011. "Spatio-Therapeutics: Drug Treatment Courts and Urban Space." *Social & Legal Studies* 20 (2): 157–172.

Moore, Kelly E., Walter Roberts, Holly H. Reid, Kathryn M. Z. Smith, Lindsay M. S. Oberleitner, and Sherry A. McKee. 2019. "Effectiveness of Medication Assisted Treatment for Opioid Use in Prison and Jail Settings: A Meta-Analysis and Systematic Review." *Journal of Substance Abuse Treatment* 99:32–43.

Morris, Monique. 2016. *Pushout: The Criminalization of Black Girls in Schools*. New Press.

Morrison, Toni. 1993. *Playing in the Dark: Whiteness And the Literary Imagination*. Vintage.

Moynihan, Daniel Patrick. 1965. "The Negro Family: The Case for National Action." US Department of Labor. www.dol.gov.

Muhuri, Pradip K., J. C. Gfroerer, and C. Davies. 2013. "Associations of Nonmedical Pain Reliever Use and Initiation of Heroin Use in the United States." Center for Behavioral Health Statistics and Quality. www.samhsa.gov.

Murphy, Jennifer. 2015. *Illness or Deviance: Drug Courts, Drug Treatment, and the Ambiguity of Addiction*. Temple University Press.

Murray, Charles. 2012. *Coming Apart: The State of White America, 1960–2010*. Crown Forum.

Musto, David F. 1999. *The American Disease: Origins of Narcotics Control*. 3rd ed. Oxford University Press.

National Park Service. 2017. "New York State Inebriate Asylum." www.nps.gov.

National Sheriffs' Association and National Commission on Correctional Health Care. 2018. "Jail-Based Medication-Assisted Treatment: Promising Practices, Guidelines, and Resources for the Field." www.sheriffs.org.

National Treatment Court Resource Center. 2024. "What Are Drug Courts?" October 25. https://ntcrc.org.

Native Land Digital. n.d. "Native Land Digital." Accessed February 8, 2025. https://native-land.ca.

Neocleous, Mark. 2003. *Imagining the State*. Open University Press.

Neocleous, Mark. 2014. *War Power, Police Power*. Edinburgh University Press.

Neocleous, Mark. 2016. *The Universal Adversary: Security, Capital and the "Enemies of All Mankind."* Routledge.

Neocleous, Mark. 2021. *The Fabrication of Social Order: A Critical Theory of Police Power*. Verso Books.

Netherland, Jules. 2023. "Good Samaritans in the War on Drugs That Wasn't." In *Whiteout: How Racial Capitalism Changed the Color of Opioids in America*, edited by Helena Hansen, Jules Netherland, and David Herzberg. University of California Press.

Netherland, Jules, and Helena Hansen. 2016. "The War on Drugs That Wasn't: Wasted Whiteness, 'Dirty Doctors,' and Race in Media Coverage of Prescription Opioid Misuse." *Culture, Medicine, and Psychiatry* 40 (4): 664–686.

New York Heritage. n.d. "Broome County Poor Farm." Empire State Library Network. Accessed October 23, 2024. https://nyheritage.org.

New York Times. 1908. "6,000 Opium Users Here." August 1.

New York Times. 1927. "Mexican Family Go Insane." July 6.

Newman, Simon. 2017. "180th Anniversary for Former Slave James McCune Smith." University of Glasgow, April 27. www.gla.ac.uk.

NIAAA (National Institute on Alcohol Abuse and Alcoholism). 2024. "Alcohol Related Emergences and Death in the United States." www.niaaa.nih.gov.

Nicosia, Nancy, John M. MacDonald, and Jeremy Arkes. 2013. "Disparities in Criminal Court Referrals to Drug Treatment and Prison for Minority Men." *American Journal of Public Health* 103 (6): 77–88.

NIDA (National Institute on Drug Abuse). 2007. "Drugs, Brains, and Behavior: The Science of Addiction." April. www.drugabuse.gov.

NIDA (National Institute on Drug Abuse). 2018. "Comorbidity: Substance Use and Other Mental Disorders." August 15. www.drugabuse.gov.

NIDA (National Institute on Drug Abuse). 2019. "Opioid Overdose Crisis." January. www.drugabuse.gov.

NIDA (National Institute on Drug Abuse). 2020. "Drug Misuse and Addiction." July. https://nida.nih.gov.

NIH (National Institutes of Health). 2018. "Health Research and Development to Stem the Opioid Crisis." October. www.nih.gov.

NIJ (National Institute of Justice). n.d. "Recidivism." Accessed November 5, 2024. https://nij.ojp.gov.

Nolan, James L. 2001. *Reinventing Justice: The American Drug Court Movement*. Princeton University Press.

Norris, Spencer. 2023a. "As New York Boosts Residential Treatment, Regulators Turn a Blind Eye to Conditions." *New York Focus*, July 18. https://nysfocus.com.

Norris, Spencer. 2023b. "'Doom County Jail': Dysfunction Plagues Program for Incarcerated Opioid Users." *New York Focus*, September 27. https://nysfocus.com.

Norris, Spencer. 2023c. "New York Mandates Peer Support in Jails, but Lets Sheriffs Keep Peers Out." *New York Focus*, May 31. https://nysfocus.com.

Norris, Spencer. 2023d. "New York Sheriffs Tried to Kill Jail Opioid Treatment Law." *New York Focus*, October 12. https://nysfocus.com.

Norton, Jack. 2018. "No One Is Watching: Jail in Upstate New York." Vera Institute of Justice, April 19. www.vera.org.

Norton, Jack. 2019. "We Are Not Going to Rest: Organizing Against Incarceration in Upstate New York." Vera Institute of Justice, September 3. www.vera.org.

Norton, Jack, Lydia Pelot-Hobbs, and Judah Schept. 2024a. "Federal Courts, FEMA Dollars, and Local Elections in the Struggle Against Phase III in New Orleans: An Interview with Lexi Peterson-Burge of Orleans Parish Prison Reform Coalition." In *The Jail Is Everywhere: Fighting the New Geography of Mass Incarceration*, edited by Jack Norton, Lydia Pelot-Hobbs, and Judah Schept. Verso Books.

Norton, Jack, Lydia Pelot-Hobbs, and Judah Schept. 2024b. "Introduction: The Jail Is Everywhere." In *The Jail Is Everywhere: Fighting the New Geography of Mass Incarceration*, edited by Jack Norton, Lydia Pelot-Hobbs, and Judah Schept. Verso Books.

Novak, Daniel A. 2014. *The Wheel of Servitude: Black Forced Labor After Slavery*. University Press of Kentucky.

NYCLU (New York Civil Liberties Union). 2022. "Protect Trans New Yorkers in Jails and Prisons." March 23. www.nyclu.org.

NYCLU (New York Civil Liberties Union). 2023. "Transgender Woman Reaches Landmark Settlement with Broome County Following Lawsuit over Discrimination, Abuse and Denial of Medical Care." August 24. www.nyclu.org.

NYS (New York State). 2021. "Governor Hochul Signs Legislation Package to Combat Opioid Crisis." October 7. www.governor.ny.gov.

NYS (New York State). n.d.-a. "Apply for SNAP." Accessed January 31, 2025. www.ny.gov.

NYS (New York State). n.d.-b. "Re-entry Able Program." NY Connects. Accessed October 22, 2024. www.nyconnects.ny.gov.

NYS Comptroller (New York State Office of the Comptroller). 2017. "Facility Oversight and Timeliness of Response to Complaints and Inmate Grievances." Division of State Government Accountability. www.osc.state.ny.us.

NYS Comptroller (New York State Office of the Comptroller). 2022. "Continuing Crisis: Drug Overdose Deaths in New York." www.osc.state.ny.us.

NYS Comptroller (New York State Office of the Comptroller). 2024. "New Yorkers in Need: The Housing Insecurity Crisis." www.osc.state.ny.us.

NYS DCJS (New York State Division of Criminal Justice Services). n.d. "New York State Index Crime." Accessed February 19, 2025. www.criminaljustice.ny.gov.

NYS DOH (New York State Department of Health). 2018. "New York State Opioid Annual Data Report 2018." www.health.ny.gov.

NYS DOH (New York State Department of Health). 2021. "New York State's 911 Good Samaritan Law Protects YOU." April. www.health.ny.gov.

NYS DOH (New York State Department of Health). 2024a. "Best Practice for the Implementation Of Buprenorphine for the Treatment of Opioid Use Disorder (OUD) from the New York State Department Of Health (DOH) and the Office of Addiction Services and Supports (OASAS)." February. www.health.ny.gov/.

NYS DOH (New York State Department of Health). 2024b. "New York State Opioid Data Dashboard." April. https://apps.health.ny.gov.

NYS OAG (New York State Office of the Attorney General). 2017. "A.G. Schneiderman Announces 39 Guilty Pleas as Part of Operation Bricktown in Syracuse." September 18. https://ag.ny.gov.

NYS OTDA (New York State Office of Temporary and Disability Assistance). 2011. "Temporary Assistance Source Book." https://otda.ny.gov.

NYS Senate (New York State Senate). 2014. "Public Forum: Monroe County. Panel Discussion on Rochester's Heroin Epidemic." The New York State Senate Majority Coalition Joint Task Force on Heroin and Opioid Addiction. April 15. www.nysenate.gov.

NYS Senate (New York State Senate). 2016. "NYS Joint Senate Task Force on Heroin and Opioid Addiction Report." May 17. www.nysenate.gov.

NYS Senate (New York State Senate). 2018. "Sen. Akshar Announces State Funding for Jail-Based Substance Use Disorder Treatment Services at the Broome County Jail." July 28. www.nysenate.gov.

NYS Senate (New York State Senate). 2021. "Section 202. 78. Witness or Victim of Drug or Alcohol Overdose." April 2. www.nysenate.gov.

NYS Senate (New York State Senate). n.d. "Article 220: Controlled Substances Offenses." Accessed February 9, 2025. www.nysenate.gov.

NYS UCS (New York State Unified Court System). n.d.-a. "Behind the Scenes of Drug Court." 6 JD Broome County. Accessed January 30, 2025. ww2.nycourts.gov.

NYS UCS (New York State Unified Court System). n.d.-b. "Broome County Drug Court." Accessed February 1, 2025. ww2.nycourts.gov.

NYS UCS (New York State Unified Court System). n.d.-c. "Drug Court Participant's Handbook." Accessed January 30, 2025. ww2.nycourts.gov.

NYS UCS (New York State Unified Court System). n.d.-d. "Drug Treatment Courts." Problem-Solving Courts. Accessed January 30, 2025. ww2.nycourts.gov.

Nyx, Eris, and Jeremy Kalicum. 2024. "A Case Study of the DULF Compassion Club and Fulfillment Centre—A Logical Step Forward in Harm Reduction." International Journal of Drug Policy 131:104537.

Oberholtzer, Elliot. 2017. "The Dismal State of Transgender Incarceration Policies." Prison Policy Initiative. www.prisonpolicy.org.

O'Brien, Rebecca Davis. 2013. "The Grim Life of Suburban Addicts." The Record, May 6.

O'Donovan, Maria. 2014. "A Tale of One City: Creative Destruction, Spatial Fixes, and Ideology in Binghamton, New York." International Journal of Historical Archaeology 18 (2): 284–298.

O'Donovan, Maria. 2019. "Nostalgia and Heritage in the Carousal City: Deindustrialization, Critical Memory, and the Future." Journal of Community Archaeology & Heritage 6 (4): 272–282.

ONDCP (Office of National Drug Control Policy). 2013. "What Drug Policy Reform Looks Like: Director's Remarks at the National Press Club." April 17. https://obamawhitehouse.archives.gov.

O'Neill, Savannah, and Eliza Wheeler. 2017. "Myths and Misinformation About Law Enforcement and Fentanyl Exposure." National Harm Reduction Coalition. https://harmreduction.org.

Ornstein, Charles, and Tracy Weber. 2012. "American Pain Foundation Shuts Down as Senators Launch Investigation of Prescription Narcotics." May 8. www.propublica.org.

Owens, Deirdre Cooper. 2022. "The Fugitive Slave Act." In *Four Hundred Souls: A Community History of African America, 1619–2019*, edited by Ibram X. Kendi and Keisha N. Blain. One World.

PAARI (Police Assisted Addiction Recovery Initiative). 2015. "Broome County, N.Y. Joins with P.A.A.R.I., Will Create Addiction Outreach and Referral Program." September 2. https://paariusa.org.

PAARI (Police Assisted Addiction Recovery Initiative). 2016a. "Broome County, N.Y. District Attorney's Office Joins P.A.A.R.I., Launches Operation S.A.F.E." February 8. https://paariusa.org.

PAARI (Police Assisted Addiction Recovery Initiative). 2016b. "Broome County, N.Y. Joins with P.A.A.R.I., Will Create Addiction Outreach and Referral Program." September 2. https://paariusa.org.

PAARI (Police Assisted Addiction Recovery Initiative). n.d.-a. "About Us." Accessed May 4, 2024. https://paariusa.org.

PAARI (Police Assisted Addiction Recovery Initiative). n.d.-b. "Our Public Safety and Community Partners." Accessed May 4, 2024. https://paariusa.org.

Page, Cara, and Erica Woodland. 2023. Conclusion to *Healing Justice Lineages: Dreaming at the Crossroads of Liberation, Collective Care, and Safety*, edited by Cara Page and Erica Woodland. North Atlantic Books.

Palmer, Chris. 2020. "Philly Police: Cop's Body Camera Caught His Punch on Apparently Overdosing Man Who Died." *Philadelphia Inquirer*, February 14. www.inquirer.com.

Patterson, Evelyn. 2013. "The Broome County Almshouse." https://digitalprojects.binghamton.edu.

Patterson, Orlando. (1982) 2018. *Slavery and Social Death: A Comparative Study*. Harvard University Press.

PDAPS (Prescription Drug Abuse Policy System). 2019. "Drug Induced Homicide Laws." *Health In Justice Action and Legal Science*. January 1. https://pdaps.org.

Penn, Andrew. 2019. "Are Benzodiazepines the Next Opioid Crisis?" *Psychiatry & Behavioral Health Learning Network*, February 19. www.psychcongress.com.

Perez, Stephen. 2019. "A Repository of Social Ills: Mass Incarceration in Broome County." The Contemporary Group, March 29. https://thecontemporarygroup.com.

Petersen, Amanda M. 2024. "Community-Oriented Copaganda: Anti-Black Violence in a Visual Archive of Policing." *Crime, Media, Culture*, February 14, 1–23.

Pew Charitable Trust. 2023. "Number of U.S. Adults on Probation or Parole Continues to Decline." October 14. www.pewtrusts.org.

Pleus, Alexis, and Kevin Revier. 2017. "Law Enforcement's Facebook Posts Promote Racism in Opioid Epidemic." *Press & Sun-Bulletin*, November 5, A1.

Pleus, Alexis, and Kevin Revier. 2018. "Skepticism over Jail Treatment Plan." *Press & Sun-Bulletin*, July 29, A1.

Porter, Dorothy. 1999. *Health, Civilization, and the State: A History of Public Health from Ancient to Modern Times*. Routledge.

Porter, Jane, and Hershel Jick. 1980. "Addiction Rare in Patients Treated with Narcotics." *New England Journal of Medicine* 302 (2): 123.

Potawatomi Nation. 2021. "Disproportionate Representation of Native Americans in Foster Care Across United States." April 6. www.potawatomi.org.

Poulantzas, Nicos. 2014. *State, Power, Socialism*. Verso.

Powell, John A. 2022. "Dred Scott." In *Four Hundred Souls: A Community History of African America, 1619–2019*, edited by Ibram X. Kendi and Keisha N. Blain. One World.

PPI (Prison Policy Initiative). 2024. "Addicted to Punishment: Jails and Prisons Punish Drug Use Far More than They Treat It." January 30. www.prisonpolicy.org.

Pragacz, Andrew J. 2016. "Is This What Decarceration Looks Like? Rising Jail Expansion in Upstate New York." In *After Prisons? Freedom, Decarceration, and Justice Disinvestment*, edited by William G. Martin and Joshua M. Price. Lexington Books.

Pragacz, Andrew J., and Kevin Revier. 2024. "'Not One More Dollar Goes into This Jail': Becoming Abolitionists in Upstate New York." In *The Jail Is Everywhere: Fighting the New Geography of Mass Incarceration*, edited by Jack Norton, Lydia Pelot-Hobbs, and Judah Schept. Verso Books.

Preble, Edward, and John J. Casey. 1969. "Taking Care of Business—the Heroin User's Life on the Street." *International Journal of the Addictions* 4 (1): 1–24.

Presdee, Mike. 2000. *Cultural Criminology and the Carnival of Crime*. Routledge.

Presser, Lois. 2016. "Criminology and the Narrative Turn." *Crime Media Culture* 12 (2): 137–151.

Price, Joshua M. 2015a. *Prison and Social Death*. Rutgers University Press.

Price, Joshua M. 2015b. "Reducing the US Prison Population Is but a Small Step." *Aeon*. https://aeon.co.

Price, Joshua M. 2016. "Serving Two Masters? Reentry Task Forces and Justice Disinvestment." In *After Prisons? Freedom, Decarceration, and Justice Disinvestment*, edited by William G. Martin and Joshua M. Price. Lexington Books.

Price, Joshua M. 2017. "Psychic Investment in Cruelty: Three Parables on Race and Imprisoning the Mentally Ill." *Contemporary Justice Review* 20 (4): 491–504.

Pride and Joy Families. n.d. "Who We Are." Accessed January 30, 2025. www.binghamton.edu.

Pruitt, Lisa R. 2019. "What *Hillbilly Elegy* Reveals About Race in Twenty-First-Century America." In *Appalachian Reckoning: A Region Responds to "Hillbilly Elegy,"* edited by Meredith McCarroll and Anthony Harkins. West Virginia University Press.

Punch, Alexandra, Mariah Brennan, and Shannon Monnat. 2022. "An Evaluation of New York State Opioid Courts: Fidelity to the 10 Essential Elements of Opioid Intervention Courts." Syracuse University Lerner Center for Public Health Promotion and Population Health.

Punch, Samantha. 2012. "Hidden Struggles of Fieldwork: Exploring the Role and Use of Field Diaries." *Emotion, Space and Society* 5 (2): 86–93.

Purnell, Derecka. 2021. *Becoming Abolitionists: Police, Protests, and the Pursuit of Freedom*. Astra.

Purser, Gretchen. 2021. "'You Put Up with Anything': On the Vulnerability and Exploitability of Formerly Incarcerated Workers." *Labor and Punishment: Work in and out of Prison*, edited by Erin Hatton. University of California Press.

Quinones, Sam. 2015. *Dreamland: The True Tail of America's Opiate Epidemic*. Bloomsbury.

Quinones, Sam. 2017. "Addicts Need Help. Jails Could Have the Answer." *New York Times*, June 16. www.nytimes.com.

Quinones, Sam. 2021. *The Least of Us: True Tales of America and Hope in the Time of Fentanyl and Meth*. Bloomsbury.

Raffo, Susan. 2023. "We Move in Relationship: Sites of Practice in the Midwest." In *Healing Justice Lineages: Dreaming at the Crossroads of Liberation, Collective Care, and Safety*, edited by Cara Page and Erica Woodland. North Atlantic Books.

Ranapurwala, Shabbar I., Meghan E. Shanahan, Apostolos A. Alexandridis, Scott K. Proescholdbell, Rebecca B. Naumann, Daniel Edwards Jr., and Stephen W. Marshall. 2018. "Opioid Overdose Mortality Among Former North Carolina Inmates: 2000–2015." *American Journal of Public Health* 108 (9): 1207–1213.

Razack, Sherene H. 2020. "Settler Colonialism, Policing and Racial Terror: The Police Shooting of Loreal Tsingine." *Feminist Legal Studies* 28 (1): 1–20.

Reding, Nick. 2010. *Methland: The Death and Life of an American Small Town*. Bloomsbury.

Reilly, Steve. 2014. "Broome Jail Inmate Death Leads to $62K Settlement." *Pressconnects*, September 12. www.pressconnects.com.

Reinarman, Craig. 1994. "The Social Construction of Drug Scares." In *Constructions of Deviance: Social Power, Context, and Interaction*, edited by Patricia Adler and Peter Adler. Nelson Education.

Reinarman, Craig. 2005. "Addiction as Accomplishment: The Discursive Construction of Disease." *Addiction Research and Theory* 13 (4): 307–320.

Reinarman, Craig, and Ceres Duskin. 1992. "Dominant Ideology and Drugs in the Media." *International Journal of Drug Policy* 3 (1): 6–15.

Reinarman, Craig, and Robert Granfield. 2014. In "Addiction Is Not Just a Brain Disease: Critical Studies of Addiction." In *Expanding Addiction: Critical Essays*, edited by Robert Granfield and Craig Reinarman. Routledge.

Reinarman, Craig, and Harry G. Levine. 1997. *Crack in America: Demon Drugs and Social Justice*. University of California Press.

Reinarman, Craig, and Harry G. Levine. 2004. "Crack in the Rearview Mirror: Deconstructing Drug War Mythology." *Social Justice* 31 (1–2): 182–199.

Reinhart, Christopher. n.d. "New York Drug Possession and Sale Crimes." Old Research Report, Connecticut General Assembly. Accessed February 9, 2025. www.cga.ct.gov.

Revier, Kevin. 2018. "'Once Again, a Meth Lab Exploded and Somebody Died': Narratives of Volatility and Risk in the Rural Drug War." *Crime, Media, Culture* 14 (3): 467–484.

Revier, Kevin. 2020a. "'A Life Lived': Collective Memory and White Racial Framing in Digital Opioid Overdose Obituaries." *Contemporary Drug Problems* 47 (4): 320–337.

Revier, Kevin. 2020b. "'Now You're Connected': Carceral Visuality and Police Power on Mobilepatrol." *Theoretical Criminology* 24 (2): 314–334.

Revier, Kevin. 2021a. "'Without Drug Court, You'll End Up in Prison or Dead': Therapeutic Surveillance and Addiction Narratives in Treatment Court." *Critical Criminology* 29 (4): 915–930.

Revier, Kevin. 2021b. "'The 'Worst of the Worst': Punitive Justice Frames in Criminal Sentencing Clips on YouTube." *Contemporary Justice Review* 24 (4): 436–456.

Revier, Kevin. 2022. "Figuring Things Out: Contemplating Drug Addiction and Disclosure in and out of the Field." *Contemporary Drug Problems* 49 (3): 319–335.

Revier, Kevin. 2023. "Carceral Behavioral Therapy: Creating the Criminal-Addict in Prison Evidence-Based Recovery Treatment." Contemporary Drug Problems Conference, Paris.

Riback, Lindsey. 2017. "Attorney General Boosts Heroin Fight." *Press & Sun-Bulletin*, April 30. A24.

Richards, Louise G. 1981. "Demographic Trends and Drug Abuse, 1980-1995." *National Institute on Drug Abuse Research Monograph* 35:1–102.

Riley, Jack. 2019. *Drug Warrior: Inside the Hunt for El Chapo and the Rise of America's Opioid Crisis*. Hachette Books.

Rios, Victor M. 2011. *Punished: Policing the Lives of Black and Latino Boys*. New York University Press.

Roberts, Dorothy. 2022. *Torn Apart: How the Child Welfare System Destroys Black Families—and How Abolition Can Build a Safer World*. Basic Books.

Robinson, Cedric J. 2020. *Black Marxism: The Making of the Black Radical Tradition*. 3rd ed. University of North Carolina Press.

Roby, John R. 2015. "Broome Plans 13 Deputies for Jail." *Press & Sun-Bulletin*, September 28, A1.

Roby, John R. 2016a. "Addiction Event Looks to Solutions." *Press & Sun-Bulletin*, May 24, A5.

Roby, John R. 2016b. "Indictments, Treatment Follow Large Drug Sweep." *Press & Sun-Bulletin*, August 4, A5.

Roby, John R. 2016c. "Lawsuit: Neglect Led to Broome Inmate's Death." *Pressconnects*, June 10. www.pressconnects.com.

Roby, John R. 2016d. "24 Addicts Up for Treatment, DA Says." *Pressconnects*, February 22. www.pressconnects.com.

Roby, John R. 2017. "Survey Finds Barriers to Opioid Treatment in Broome." *Pressconnects*, February 23. www.pressconnects.com.

Rodolico, Jack. 2016. "Anatomy of Addiction: How Heroin and Opioids Hijack the Brain." *NPR*, January 11. www.npr.org.

Room, Robin. 2003. "The Culture Framing of Addiction." *Janus Head* 6 (2): 221–234.

Rosenberg, Alana, Allison K. Groves, and Kim M. Blankenship. 2017. "Comparing Black and White Drug Offenders: Implications for Racial Disparities in Criminal Justice and Reentry Policy and Programming." *Journal of Drug Issues* 47 (1): 132–142.

Rosenberg, Charles. 1989. "Disease in History: Frames and Framers." *Milbank Quarterly* 67 (1): 1–15.

Ross, Luana. 1998. *Inventing the Savage: The Social Construction of Native American Criminality*. University of Texas Press.

Ross, Luana. 2004. "Native Women, Mean-Spirited Drugs, and Punishing Policies." *Social Justice* 31 (4): 54–62.

Rothman, David J. 2017. *Conscience and Convenience: The Asylum and Its Alternatives in Progressive America*. 2nd ed. Routledge.

Rubin, Jay L. 2016. *The Forgotten Kapital: The Ku Klux Klan in Binghamton, New York, 1923–1928*. Bundy Museum Press.

Rubio-Ramos, Melissa. 2022. "From Plantations to Prisons: The Race Gap in Incarceration after the Abolition of Slavery in the US." ECONtribute Discussion Paper 195.

Ruhm, Christopher J. 2022. "Living and Dying in America: An Essay on *Deaths of Despair and the Future of Capitalism*." *Journal of Economic Literature* 60 (4): 1159–1187.

Rush, Benjamin. 1784. *An Inquiry in the Effects of Ardent Spirits on the Human Body and Mind*. James Loring.

Rush, Benjamin. 1812. *Medical Inquiries and Observations, upon the Diseases of the Mind*. Kimber and Richardson.

Russell, Emma K., Bree Carlton, and Danielle Tyson. 2022. "Carceral Churn: A Sensorial Ethnography of the Bail and Remand Court." *Punishment & Society* 24 (2): 151–169.

Russell, Jessie. 2018. "Laree's Law Would Allow Police to Charge Drug Dealers with Homicide in the Case of an Overdose." *Legislative Gazette*, March 26. https://legislativegazette.com.

Sacco, Lisa N. 2018. "Federal Support for Drug Courts: In Brief." Congressional Research Service. https://sgp.fas.org.

Sack, David. 2018. "Will Adderall Be the New Opioid Crisis?" *Psychology Today*, May 22. www.psychologytoday.com.

Saleh-Hanna, Viviane. 2015. "Black Feminist Hauntology. Rememory the Ghosts of Abolition?" *Champ Pénal / Penal Field* 12. http://champpenal.revues.org.

Salinas, Mike. 2023. "'Doubling Up': Drug Dealing as a Profitable Side-Hustle." In *Understanding Drug Dealing and Illicit Drug Markets: National and International Perspectives*, edited by Tammy C. Ayres and Craig Ancrum. Routledge.

Samaritan Daytop Village. n.d. "Intensive Residential Treatment." Accessed January 30, 2025. www.samaritanvillage.org.

SAMHSA (Substance Use and Mental Health Service Administration). 2011. "Results from the 2010 National Survey on Drug Use and Health: A Summary of National Findings." www.samhsa.gov.

SAMHSA (Substance Use and Mental Health Service Administration). 2015. "Results from the 2014 National Survey on Drug Use and Health: Detailed Tables." Center for Behavior Health Statistics and Quality. www.samhsa.gov.

SAMHSA (Substance Use and Mental Health Service Administration). 2016. "SAMHSA's Working Definition of Recovery: Ten Guiding Principles of Recovery." www.samhsa.gov.

SAMHSA (Substance Use and Mental Health Service Administration). 2024. "Co-occurring Disorders and Other Health Conditions." March 29. www.samhsa.gov.

Samson, Sara. 2017. "Protesters Voice Support for Jail Alternatives at Meeting of Cortland County Legislators." *Cortland Voice*, December 1. https://cortlandvoice.com.

Sandberg, Sveinung, and Heith Copes. 2013. "Speaking with Ethnographers: The Challenges of Researching Drug Dealers and Offenders." *Journal of Drug Issues* 43 (2): 176–197.

Santos, Boaventura de Sousa. 2007. "Beyond Abyssal Thinking: From Global Lines to Ecologies of Knowledge." *Review Fernand Braudel Center* 30 (1): 45–89.

Sarai, Tamar. 2024. "'One Million Experiments' Showcases Liberatory Future-Building on a Micro Scale." *Prism*, February 26. https://prismreports.org.

Schenwar, Maya, and Victoria Law. 2020. *Prison by Any Other Name: The Harmful Consequences of Popular Reforms*. New Press.

Schept, Judah. 2012. "Contesting the 'Justice Campus': Abolitionist Resistance to Liberal Carceral Expansion." *Radical Criminology* 1 (1):37–66.

Schept, Judah. 2014. "(Un)Seeing like a Prison: Counter-Visual Ethnography of the Carceral State." *Theoretical Criminology* 18 (2): 198–223.

Schept, Judah. 2015. *Progressive Punishment: Job Loss, Growth, and the Neoliberal Logic of Carceral Expansion*. New York University Press.

Schept, Judah. 2022. *Coals Cages Crisis: The Rise of the Prison Economy in Central Appalachia*. New York University Press.

Schneider, Joseph W. 1978. "Deviant Drinking as Disease: Alcoholism as a Social Accomplishment." *Social Problems* 25 (4): 361–372.

Schofield, Daisy. 2024. "'It Could Be the Next Opioid Crisis': The Author Warning the World About Ozempic." *GQ*, May 1. www.gq-magazine.co.uk.

Schwartz, Yardena. 2012. "Painkiller Use Breeds New Face of Heroin Addiction." *NBC News*, June 29. www.hcdrugfree.org.

Schwarz, Hannah. 2017. "Program to Help Opioid Users Not as Advertised." *Press & Sun Bulletin*, May 3, A2.

Scott, Rebecca. 2010. *Removing Mountains: Extracting Nature and Identity in the Appalachian Coalfields*. University of Minnesota Press.

Seear, Kate, and Suzanne Fraser. 2010. "Ben Cousins and the 'Double Life': Exploring Citizenship and the Voluntary/Compulsivity Binary Through the Experiences of a 'Drug Addicted' Elite Athlete." *Critical Public Health* 20 (4): 439–452.

Seelye, Katherine. 2015. "In Heroin Crisis, White Families Seek Gentler War on Drugs." *New York Times*, October 30. www.nytimes.com.

Seigel, Micol. 2018. *Violence Work: State Power and the Limits of Police*. Duke University Press.

Seward, William Foote. 1924. *Binghamton and Broome County: A History*. Lewis Historical.

Shay, Jack Edward. 2012. *Bygone Binghamton: Remembering People and Places of the Past*. Vol. 1. AuthorHouse.

Sheff, David. 2013. *Clean: Overcoming Addiction and Ending America's Greatest Tragedy*. Houghton Mifflin Harcourt.

Simon, Jonathan. 2001. "Governing Through Crime Metaphors." *Brooklyn Law Review* 67 (4): 1035–1070.

Singhal, Astha, Yu-Yu Tien, and Renee Y. Hsia. 2016. "Racial-Ethnic Disparities in Opioid Prescriptions at Emergency Department Visits for Conditions Commonly Associated with Prescription Drug Abuse." *PLOS ONE* 11 (8): 1–14.

Sinha, Shreeya. 2018. "Heroin Addiction Explained: How Opioids Hijack the Brain." *New York Times*, December 18. www.nytimes.com.

Skelos, Dean G. 2011. "Senate Gives Final Legislative Approval to 'Good Samaritan' Law." New York State Senate, June 20. www.nysenate.gov.

Smiley-McDonald, Hope M., Peyton R. Attaway, Nicholas J. Richardson, Peter J. Davidson, and Alex H. Kral. 2022. "Perspectives from Law Enforcement Officers Who Respond to Overdose Calls for Service and Administer Naloxone." *Health & Justice* 10 (1): 1–13.

Smith, Briana. 2018. "Local Organization Says Less Jail, More Treatment for Drug Users." Spectrum News 1, January 16. https://spectrumlocalnews.com.

Smith, Peter Andrey. 2018. "What Can Make a 911 Call a Felony? Fentanyl at the Scene." *New York Times*, December 17. www.nytimes.com.

Solomon, Robert. 2020. "Racism and Its Effect on Cannabis Research." *Cannabis and Cannabinoid Research* 5 (1): 2–5.

Soss, Joe, Richard C. Fording, and Sanford Schram. 2011. *Disciplining the Poor: Neoliberal Paternalism and the Persistent Power of Race*. University of Chicago Press.

Spectrum News Staff. 2016. "Suspected Drug Kingpin Arraigned." Spectrum News 1, August 11. https://spectrumlocalnews.com.

Spectrum News Staff. 2018. "State Senate Approves Plan to Add Addiction Services to Jail." Spectrum News 1, June 21. https://spectrumlocalnews.com.

Spencer, Dale. 2009. "Sex Offender as Homo Sacer." *Punishment and Society* 11 (2): 219–240.

Spencer, Merianne R., Arialdi M. Miniño, and Margaret Warner. 2022. "Drug Overdose Deaths in the United States, 2001–2021." *NCHS Data Brief* 457:1–8.

Sprout Distro. 2017. "12 Things to Do Instead of Calling the Cops." January 28. www.sproutdistro.com.

SRLP (Sylvia Rivera Law Project), PAC (Prisoner Advisory Committee), and TakeRoot (TakeRoot Justice). 2021. "It's Still War in Here. A Statewide Report on the Trans, Gender Non-Conforming, Intersex (TGNCI) Experience in New York Prisons and the Fight for Trans Liberation, Self-Determination, and Freedom." https://takeroot-justice.org.

Staff. 2016. "Operation SAFE Gets Treatment for Addicts." *Binghamton Homepage*, February 8. www.binghamtonhomepage.com.

Stanciu, Brett Ann. 2021. *Unstitched: My Journey to Understand Opioid Addiction and How People and Communities Can Heal.* Steerforth.

Stanton, Arlene, Caroline McLeod, Bill Luckey, W. B. Kissin, and L. J. Sonnefeld. 2006. "Expanding Treatment of Opioid Dependence: Initial Physician and Patient Experiences with the Adoption of Buprenorphine." Presentation at the American Society of Addiction Medicine.

Stanton, Dan. 2015. "Suboxone Sales Down as Opioid Addiction Drug Market Intensifies." *Outsourcing Pharma*, February 12. www.outsourcing-pharma.com.

Statista. 2024a. "Percentage of Violent Crimes in the United States Reported to the Police in 2023." www.statista.com.

Statista. 2024b. "Total Federal Drug Control Spending in the United States from FY 2012 to FY 2025." www.statista.com.

Stenersen, Madeline R., Kathryn Thomas, and Sherry McKee. 2024. "Police Harassment and Violence Against Transgender & Gender Diverse Sex Workers in the United States." *Journal of Homosexuality* 71 (3): 828–840.

Stevenson, Bryan. 2017. "A Presumption of Guilt." In *Policing the Black Man*, edited by Angela J. Davis. Pantheon Books.

Stöver, Heino, and Fabienne Hariga. 2016. "Prison-Based Needle and Syringe Programmes (PNSP)—Still Highly Controversial After All These Years." *Drugs: Education, Prevention and Policy* 23 (2): 103–112.

Strings, Sabrina. 2019. *Fearing the Black Body: The Racial Origins of Fat Phobia.* New York University Press.

Subramanian, Ram, Christine Riley, and Chris Mai. 2018. "Divided Justice: Trends in Black and White Jail Incarceration, 1990–2013." Vera Institute of Justice. www.vera. org.

Sullivan, Andrew. 2018. "The Poison We Pick." *New York*, February 19. https://nymag. com.

Sullivan, Mark Daniel, and Jane Ballantyne. 2023. *The Right to Pain Relief and Other Deep Roots of the Opioid Epidemic.* Oxford University Press.

Sykes, Gresham M. (1952) 2007. *The Society of Captives: A Study of a Maximum Security Prison.* Princeton University Press.

Szalavitz, Maia. 2016. *Unbroken Brain: A Revolutionary New Way of Understanding Addiction.* St. Martin's.

Talbot, Margaret. 2017. "The Addicts Next Door." *New Yorker*, June 5. www.newyorker. com.

Tastrom, Katie. 2024. *A People's Guide to Abolition and Disability Justice.* PM Press.

Tatum, Beverly Daniel. 2017. *Why Are All the Black Kids Still Sitting Together in the Cafeteria? and Other Conversations about Race in the Twenty-First Century.* Basic Books.

Taylor, Stuart. 2016. "Moving Beyond The Other: A Critique of the Reductionist Drugs Discourse." *Cultuur and Criminaliteit* 6 (1): 100–118.

Thier, Hadas. 2020. *A People's Guide to Capitalism: An Introduction to Marxist Economics*. Haymarket Books.

Tiger, Rebecca. 2011. "Drug Courts and the Logic of Coerced Treatment." *Sociological Forum* 26 (1): 169–182.

Tiger, Rebecca. 2013. *Judging Addicts: Drug Courts and Coercion in the Justice System*. New York University Press.

Town of Binghamton, New York. n.d. "About the Town of Binghamton." Accessed January 30, 2025. https://townofbinghamton.com.

Treadwell, James, and Craig Kelly. 2023. "Violence, Grime, Gangs and Drugs on the South Side of Birmingham." In *Understanding Drug Dealing and Illicit Drug Markets: National and International Perspectives*, edited by Tammy C. Ayres and Craig Ancrum. Routledge.

Tunnell, Kenneth D. 2004. "Cultural Constructions of the Hillbilly Heroin and Crime Problem." In *Cultural Criminology Unleashed*, edited by Jeff Ferrell, Keith Hayward, Wayne Morrison, and Mike Presdee. Routledge.

Turner, Justin, and Travis Milburn. 2024. "Citizen Empowerment as a Police Force Multiplier: Reproducing Social Domination Through a 21st Century Personal Safety App." *Crime, Media, Culture*, February 10.

Ugelvik, Thomas. 2014. *Power and Resistance in Prison: Doing Time, Doing Freedom*. Springer.

UPI (United Press International). 1982. "Text of President and Mrs. Reagan's Saturday Radio Address." October 2. www.upi.com.

US CBP (US Customs and Border Protection). 2024. "Drug Seizure Statistics." April 12. www.cbp.gov.

US Congress. 1970. *Controlled Dangerous Substances, Narcotics, and Drug Control Laws: Hearings Before the Committee on Ways and Means, House of Representatives, Ninety-First Congress, Second Session on Legislation to Regulate Controlled Dangerous Substances and Amend Narcotics and Drug Laws*. US Government Printing Office.

US Congress. 2018. International Narcotics Trafficking Emergency Response by Detecting Incoming Contraband with Technology (INTERDICT) Act. January 10. www.congress.gov.

US House of Representative, Committee on Oversight and Reform. 2021. "The Role of Purdue Pharma and the Sackler Family in the Opioid Epidemic." US Government Publishing Office, December 17. www.govinfo.gov.

Vakharia, Sheila P. 2024. *The Harm Reduction Gap: Helping Individuals Left Behind by Conventional Drug Prevention and Abstinence-Only Addiction Treatment*. Routledge.

Van Zee, Art. 2009. "The Promotion and Marketing of Oxycontin: Commercial Triumph, Public Health Tragedy." *American Journal of Public Health* 99 (2): 221–227.

Venters, Homer. 2019. *Life and Death in Rikers Island*. Johns Hopkins University Press.

Vera Institute of Justice. 2019. "Incarceration Trends in New York." www.vera.org.

Vera Institute of Justice. 2021. "Fast Facts: Broome County." *Empire State of Incarceration*. www.vera.org.

Vera Institute of Justice. 2023. "Broome County, NY." *Vera Incarceration Trends*, August 21. https://trends.vera.org.

Vincent, Louise. 2018. "The Rage of Overdose Grief Makes It All Too Easy to Misdirect Blame." *Filter*, December 5. https://filtermag.org.

Vincent, Louise. 2022. "I Want to Reclaim My Voice from 'Light Up the Night.'" *Filter*, January 14. https://filtermag.org.

Virey, Julien-Joseph. 1837. *Natural History of the Negro Race*. D. J. Dowling.

Vitale, Alex. 2017. *The End of Policing*. Verso Books.

Volkow, Nora D. 2014. "America's Addiction to Opioids: Heroin and Prescription Drug Abuse." National Institute on Drug Abuse, May 14. https://archives.drugabuse.gov.

Volkow, Nora D. 2015. "Addiction Is a Disease of Free Will." *National Institute on Drug Abuse Blog*, June 12.

Volkow, Nora D., and Francis Collins. 2017. "The Role of Science in Addressing the Opioid Crisis." *New England Journal of Medicine* 377 (4): 391–394.

Volkow, Nora, and Ting-Kai Li. 2005. "The Neuroscience of Addiction." *Nature Neuroscience* 8 (11): 1429–1430.

Vornik, Lana A., and E. Sherwood Brown. 2006. "Management of Comorbid Bipolar Disorder and Substance Abuse." *Journal of Clinical Psychiatry* 67 (7): 24–30.

Vrecko, Scott. 2010. "'Civilizing Technologies' and the Control of Deviance." *Biosocieties* 5 (1): 36–51.

Wakeman, Sarah E., Marc R. Larochelle, Omid Ameli, Christine E. Chaisson, Jeffrey Thomas McPheeters, William H. Crown, Francisca Azocar, and Darshak M. Sanghavi. 2020. "Comparative Effectiveness of Different Treatment Pathways for Opioid Use Disorder." *JAMA Network Open* 3 (2): 1–12.

Wakeman, Stephen. 2014. "Fieldwork, Biography and Emotion: Doing Criminological Autoethnography." *British Journal of Criminology* 54 (5): 705–721.

Walby, Kevin, Matthew Ferguson, and Justin Piché. 2020. "'Take a Look at Yourself': Digital Displays at Police Museums as Camouflage." *Annual Review of Interdisciplinary Justice Research* 9:57–85.

Walfred, Michele. 2016. "Irish Stereotype." Thomas Nast Cartoons, March 1. https://thomasnastcartoons.com.

Wall, Tyler. 2016. "Ordinary Emergency: Drones, Police, and Geographies of Legal Terror." *Antipode* 48 (4): 1122–1139.

Wall, Tyler. 2020. "The Police Invention of Humanity: Notes on the 'Thin Blue Line.'" *Crime, Media, Culture* 16 (3): 319–336.

Wall, Tyler, and Travis Linnemann. 2014. "Staring Down the State: Police Power, Visual Economies, and the 'War on Cameras.'" *Crime Media Culture* 10 (2): 133–149.

Walter, Hannah. 2019. "The Penitentiary Paradox: Carceral-Based Substance Use Treatment and Health Mismanagement." Department of Sociology, Binghamton University.

Washington, Harriet A. 2022. "James McCune Smith." In *Four Hundred Souls: A Community History of African America, 1619–2019*, edited by Ibram X. Kendi and Keisha N. Blain. One World.

Washton, Arnold. 1986. "Kids and Cocaine: An Epidemic Strikes Middle America." *Newsweek*, March 17, 58–65.

Weller, Jack E. 1965. *Yesterday's People: Life in Contemporary Appalachia*. University Press of Kentucky.

Wells, Ida B. (1892) 2013. *Southern Horrors: Lynch Law in All its Phases*. Aukland: Floating Press.

Wexler, David B., and Bruce J. Winick. 1996. *Law in a Therapeutic Key: Developments in Therapeutic Jurisprudence*. Carolina Academic Press.

White House. 2011. "Drug Courts." Office of the National Drug Control Policy (ONDCP). https://obamawhitehouse.archives.gov.

White House. 2016. "The White House." July 22. https://obamawhitehouse.archives.gov.

White House. 2018. "Remarks by President Trump on Combatting the Opioid Crisis." March 19. https://trumpwhitehouse.archives.gov.

White House. 2022a. "Fact Sheet: President Biden's Safer America Plan." August 1. www.whitehouse.gov.

White House. 2022b. "Fact Sheet: White House Releases 2022 National Drug Control Strategy That Outlines Comprehensive Path Forward to Address Addiction and the Overdose Epidemic." *Briefing Room*, April 21. www.whitehouse.gov.

White House. n.d. "The Administration's Strategy." Office of the National Drug Control Policy (ONDCP). Accessed February 1, 2025. https://trumpwhitehouse.archives.gov.

White House Council of Economic Advisors. 2019. "The Full Cost of the Opioid Crisis: $2.5 Trillion over Four Years." https://trumpwhitehouse.archives.gov.

WHO (World Health Organization). 2022. "Mental Health." June 17. www.who.int.

WHO (World Health Organization). 2023a. "Opioid Overdose." August 29. www.who.int.

WHO (World Health Organization). 2023b. "Tobacco." July 31. www.who.int.

WHO (World Health Organization). 2024. "Alcohol." June 28. www.who.int.

Whyte, Kathy. 2014. "Broome Mental Health Clinic Patients to Transfer." WNBF, June 5. https://wnbf.com.

Whyte, Kathy. 2017. "Queens Woman Accused of Supplying Cocaine and Heroin Upstate." WNBF, August 9. https://wnbf.com.

Wideman, John Edgar. (1984) 2020. *Brothers and Keepers: A Memoir*. Scribner.

Wilkerson, Albert Ernest. 1966. "A History of the Concept of Alcoholism as a Disease." PhD diss., University of Pennsylvania.

Williams, Edward Huntington. 1914. "'Negro Cocaine' Fiends Are a New Southern Menace." *New York Times*, February 8.

Williams, Kidada E. 2023. *I Saw Death Coming: A History of Terror and Survival in the War Against Reconstruction*. Bloomsbury.

Williamson, Kevin. 2016. "The Father-Führer." *National Review*, March 28. www.nationalreview.com.

Wilson, Nana. 2020. "Drug and Opioid-Involved Overdose Deaths—United States, 2017–2018." *Morbidity and Mortality Weekly Report* 69 (11): 290–297.

Wood, Ellen Meiksins. 2017. *The Origin of Capitalism: A Longer View*. Verso Books.

Woodland, Erica. 2023a. "Building the World We Want and Deserve: Sites of Practice in California." In *Healing Justice Lineages: Dreaming at the Crossroads of Liberation, Collective Care, and Safety,* edited by Cara Page and Erica Woodland. North Atlantic Books.

Woodland, Erica. 2023b. "We Are Our History: Transforming the Legacy of Criminalization." In *Healing Justice Lineages: Dreaming at the Crossroads of Liberation, Collective Care, and Safety,* edited by Cara Page and Erica Woodland. North Atlantic Books.

World Population Review. n.d. "Binghamton, New York Population 2023." Accessed February 1, 2025. https://worldpopulationreview.com.

Wray, Matt. 2006. *Not Quite White: White Trash and the Boundaries of Whiteness.* Duke University Press.

Wright, Sarah. 2016. "'Ah . . . The Power of Mothers': Bereaved Mothers as Victims-Heroes in Media Enacted Crusades for Justice." *Crime Media Culture* 12 (3): 327–343.

Wyatt, Ronald. 2013. "Pain and Ethnicity." *American Medical Association Journal of Ethics* 15 (5): 449–454.

Zahavi, Gerald. 1988. *Workers, Managers, and Welfare Capitalism: The Shoemakers and Tanners of Endicott Johnson, 1890–1950.* University of Illinois Press.

Zakaria, Fareed. 2012. "Incarceration Nation." *Time,* April 2. https://time.com.

INDEX

ABOUT THE AUTHOR

KEVIN REVIER is Assistant Professor of Criminology in the Department of Sociology/Anthropology at the State University of New York at Cortland. He is the coauthor of *America's Horror Stories: U.S. History Through Dark Tourism*. His writing has appeared in *Filter*, *Truthout*, and *CounterPunch*.